# Your Symptoms Are Real

## What to Do When Your Doctor Says Nothing Is Wrong

BENJAMIN H. NATELSON, M.D.

BICENTENNIAL
1807
WILEY
2007
BICENTENNIAL

John Wiley & Sons, Inc.

Table on page 54 © Brimacombe, et al. *Journal of Clinical Psychology in Medical Settings*, 9(4): 309–314, 2002, reproduced with permission; graph on page 58 © Zhang, et al., *Chronobiology International*, 17:95–100, 2000; diagram on page 60 © *Arthritis & Rheumatism* 1990: 33(22), reprinted with permission of Wiley-Liss, Inc., a subsidiary of John Wiley & Sons, Inc; graph on page 106 © 1999 Massachusetts Medical Society. All rights reserved; Epworth test on page 129 © MW Johns 1990–1997, reproduced with permission.

Wiley Bicentennial Logo: Richard J. Pacifico

Design and compostition by Navta Associates, Inc.

The information contained in this book is not intended to serve as a replacement for professional medical advice. Any use of the information in this book is at the reader's discretion. The author and the publisher specifically disclaim any and all liability arising directly or indirectly from the use or application of any information contained in this book. A health care professional should be consulted regarding your specific situation.

For general information about our other products and services, please contact our Customer Care Department within the United States at (800) 762-2974, outside the United States at (317) 572-3993 or fax (317) 572-4002.

Wiley also publishes its books in a variety of electronic formats. Some content that appears in print may not be available in electronic books. For more information about Wiley products, visit our web site at www.wiley.com.

ISBN: 978-0-471-74028-5

Printed in the United States of America

10  9  8  7  6  5  4  3  2  1

To academic medicine, which allowed me to grow as a person, a scholar, and a doctor, and to my family, for their love and support through all the years of that process

# Contents

PART THREE

## What Else You Need to Know

# Acknowledgments

I want to thank Dr. Lenny Jason for his input on cognitive behavioral therapy and on using the buddy system, and David Shanahoff-Khalsa for choosing Kundalini yoga exercises to help people get on the wellness path. I would also like to thank Dr. David Rapoport for his input on the chapter on sleep and Drs. Tom Findley and Karen Quigley for sharing with me their balance data shown in chapter 9. And, lastly, I thank my wife and research colleague, Dr. Gudrun Lange, for her thoughtful and patient input and encouragement throughout the many years it took for this book to become a reality.

Twenty years ago, when I was seeking direction on how to get my first book published, I managed to get Norman Cousins, the famous journalist-author, on the phone for one minute. He had three words of advice: "Get an agent!" This turned out to be easier said than done, in that making this happen took many years. But the editor of my second book, Jean Black of Yale University Press, pointed me to Sharon Hogan, who helped me prepare the proposal that led Robert Shepard to accept me as a client. I can't thank Jean and Sharon enough for this. Having Robert take me on as client opened whole new vistas of understanding for me about the publishing industry. My thanks to him for everything he did to make this book look like it does today. And finally, my thanks to Christel Winkler and Tom Miller, my editors at Wiley, for their help in moving the manuscript through the editorial process.

# Introduction

I started writing this book four years ago because of many people, just like you, who came to me and asked, "Why do I feel so awful?" or "What can be done to help me feel better?" or "I know there is something wrong with me, but my doctors tell me that there isn't." I wrote this book to try to answer those questions. I can't promise that reading this book will absolutely relieve all of your concerns and symptoms at once. But I can promise you that if you read this book and try to employ the strategies I suggest, you *will* feel better than you do at this moment, quite possibly very much better. This book will help you to better understand why you feel the way you do, and it will help you to get your doctor to help you, as well as help you to help yourself.

Do you have bone-crushing fatigue, pain that is so severe you can hardly move, or difficulty thinking and concentrating? If so, has your doctor helped you? The answer is probably not. Doctors have procedures for getting to the bottom of all kinds of symptoms. But when the doctor can't find a reason for the symptoms, then the patient may find that she is on her own with no doctor to help her or guide her. Even if her doctor knows the textbook definitions that have come to describe such illnesses as chronic fatigue syndrome, fibromyalgia, and others, he or she often does not know what to do to help relieve these problems.

When this happens, a serious disconnect between you and your doctor is seldom far behind. Your doctor becomes frustrated because he or she can't come up with an explanation for your complaints, and you become frustrated because you leave the doctor's office with no answers except perhaps a hearty, "Don't worry about it, there's nothing wrong," or, much worse and all too common, the dreaded words "It's all in your head." If you do get an answer, you may find it to be contradictory, complicated, or based on out-of-date information. People aren't stupid, and the Internet has allowed access to a great deal of medical information that was once very hard to come by. Beyond all that, if you face crushing fatigue or stabbing pain each and every day, you don't need to know much more to be sure that something is truly wrong with your body.

Unfortunately, this story is not unusual. Up to 20 percent of all patients who seek medical care, primarily women, have no easily diagnosed cause for their problems. That means literally millions of patients. I know, because more than two thousand of them have come to me when their doctors, and any number of specialists, haven't been able to come up with a diagnosis and treatment plan to reduce symptoms and improve wellness.

This problem is a major women's health issue. You may be striving to live a successful life in spite of your symptoms but are having difficulty doing so. You may be teeter-tottering at the point of leaving work on short-term or long-term disability. You may be a disabled person isolated by your illness. Although I am dedicated to trying to teach doctors how to deal with you, that process could take decades. In the meantime, I have written this book for *you*.

I've organized this book into three parts designed to reconceptualize your experience and the experiences of people who seek help for fatigue, pain, or trouble concentrating. Like many others with your problem, you have probably gone to the doctor and received the diagnosis of "nothing wrong." If you are sick enough and if your doctor is aware enough, you may have gotten the diagnosis of chronic fatigue syndrome or fibromyalgia. But chances are, despite the diagnosis, your doctor told you, "There really isn't any treatment for these problems; just try harder." If anything, that kind of "treatment" may make you feel worse, not better. So your next step is to seek advice or treatment from another doctor. This doctor shopping is very unsatisfying and leads to your having problems with the medical profession and a sense that you're on your own, which may make you feel out of control and turn you to alternative therapies. While these could prove useful in putting you onto the road back to wellness, you have to be cautious in taking this step. We live in a time when late-night television is filled with hours of commercials for potions and tablets whose value is dubious at best, if not completely worthless. Telling the good from the bad is important. The purpose of this book is to fill in these blanks in both traditional and nontraditional medicine for you, so you can start getting well.

This book offers a comprehensive, practical, and new approach to getting well: the same time-tested approach I use in my own practice. In part one I discuss you, your feelings, and your symptoms. There I give you a road map of what your doctor is thinking while evaluating you and considering about your complaints. Then I lay out the ABC's of how the medical profession thinks about your sort of problem and how the doctor adds up the facts to come to a diagnosis in some cases. The section finishes with the tools needed to navigate your way through the medical options available to you despite your diagnosis of "nothing wrong" syndrome. Specifically, I'll tell you how to interact with your doctor so that your communication can, indeed, improve. Barring that, I'll show you what you'll need to know and do to get a second opinion.

Part two is the heart of the book. I start with the issue of depression, an illness that makes all symptoms worse and can produce fatigue and pain by itself. Then I discuss what we know about stress—another factor that makes symptoms worse—and what you can do to cope with it. Next, I talk about sleep so you can understand what your sleep issues are in order to attack them. Allowing your body the rest it needs to work toward wellness is critical. Then, in the next two chapters, I offer an approach to wellness that starts with medicines and then goes on to ways you can participate in the wellness process through gentle exercise.

Finally, in part three, I lay out some more complementary approaches to becoming well. Then I explain how alternative medicine can slide down into quackery. The book ends with a careful look at cutting-edge research aimed to better understand debilitating symptoms and some promising treatments that are already on the horizon.

My approach to illness has been shaped by my interaction with patients. So I often use patient stories to make points in the book. Rest assured that I have changed all patient names to ensure confidentiality.

PART ONE

# SYMPTOMS, SIGNS, SYNDROMES, AND ILLNESS

The Path to Understanding
Why You Feel Sick

# 1

# You, Your Symptoms, and Your Doctor

Sarah Jones, a thirty-four-year-old married lawyer with no children and a busy professional and social life, visited my office complaining of progressive fatigue. Her lack of energy had become so severe that she was forced to cut way back on her activities. Yet, because she'd always seemed so full of nervous energy, Mrs. Jones's doctor dismissed her complaints, telling her she was just a worrier who focused too much on how she felt. Simply put, there was "nothing wrong" with her.

## Symptoms, Illness, and Disease

When you don't feel well, it's normal to worry about what might be wrong. When the connection is clear and the problem not so bad, you may cope with the problem by yourself. For example, if your ankle becomes swollen and painful after you take a misstep and twist it, you might try to treat it yourself by putting on an elastic bandage and taking some ibuprofen. But if it hurts to stand on the ankle and you fear that the problem is worse than a minor twist, you may decide that you need medical care and go to see a doctor. The moment you seek medical care, you become a patient.

Some of the things that make people seek medical attention are fairly typical, while others are unique to specific personal characteristics. Seeking medical help if you're well one moment and in obvious trouble the next—for instance, if a bloody nose fails to stop bleeding or abdominal cramps go from trivial to awful in the course of a few hours—is a no-brainer. But when problems develop gradually, all bets are off. When I was a medical intern, I was called to the emergency room to admit a sixty-year-old woman with a seventy-five-inch waist. Why, I asked, did the family wait until that day to bring her in for medical attention. The answer was simple: "She got so big she could not get out of bed by herself." The medical evaluation was completed in a day or two and revealed an enormous ovarian tumor.

You'll probably find the family's answer to my question jarring. I know I did. How, you will ask, could the patient and her family not have known that something was wrong? The answer is that illness recognition and the decision to seek medical help are very personal issues. Medical sociologists have made this a point for study. Low socioeconomic status and poverty are two factors preventing many people from seeking medical attention until they can no longer get to their feet. Gender is another factor. The popular medical press is full of stories of men attributing their crushing chest pain to indigestion, often with fatal consequences. Women, statistics show, are more health conscious, more attuned to their bodies, and more willing to ask professional opinions about why they feel the way they do.

The question of who seeks medical attention, and when, gets murkier when an individual just feels lousy. Symptoms are the sensations that make a person feel unwell; they may bother, annoy, or hurt you. Neither the person with the bloody nose nor the woman with the enormous girth had any symptoms; instead, they had obvious abnormalities. When a person goes to the doctor feeling unwell, she reports how she feels to the doctor. The doctor then examines the patient and tries to find abnormalities that would indicate some underlying disease process. These are signs. So bleeding from the nose or having an enormous waist circumference are signs of a medical problem. For example, the patient with the twisted ankle will complain of the symptom of pain and the doctor will detect signs of the traumatic event, in the form of swelling and an area of black-and-blue skin reflecting a hemorrhage beneath the skin.

With the nose bleed, there really are no symptoms, just the evidence of blood coming from the nose. If the hemorrhage were in the stomach and not in the nose, the patient might eventually develop the symptom of lightheadedness when he or she stood up. This would occur because the gradual loss of blood into the stomach would reduce the volume of blood in the circulation, leaving insufficient blood for the brain at the moment the person stood up. Here the doctor would have to find the sign of underlying disease—either pressure-induced tenderness in the stomach suggestive of an ulcer or a positive test for blood in the stool.

When the doctor can connect the symptom with some sign, he or she is on the way to the diagnosis of a disease. If an otherwise well, middle-aged woman complains to her doctor of dizziness when she stands and a feeling of gnawing pain in her abdomen after eating, the doctor may think of the possibility of a bleeding ulcer. Finding blood in the stool makes the doctor quite sure of the diagnosis. But in order to clinch the diagnosis, the doctor will have to order a test to visualize the gut, either by X-ray or by direct observation using a flexible tool called an endoscope. When the ulcer is seen, the logic chain ends with a diagnosis: a bleeding ulcer.

One way of understanding what is meant by the term *disease* is to think of it as an all-or-nothing idea: either you have a disease or you don't. A healthy person would not have a touch of cancer; instead, the person goes from being healthy to having cancer. Although this is a bit of a simplification—precancerous conditions do indeed exist and are common—this all-or-nothing idea still helps us to understand the difference between disease and illness. In the greater scheme of things, disease is uncommon, while illness is extremely common. When a person has symptoms, she feels ill; that is, she has an illness. So while you probably have no idea what it is like to experience cancer, you have certainly experienced symptoms like pain that was there one day and not another. A temporary headache or a bellyache is a symptom, and so is severe, exhausting fatigue.

Sometimes, symptoms can be explained easily; maybe you partied too much the night before you experienced feelings of achiness or of exhaustion. Going to bed very late while still waking up at 7 a.m. is a common cause of fatigue. A day of vigorous physical activity without months of preparation at the gym is another common cause of achiness and fatigue. That's what bed rest and aspirin are for. But when your symptoms go on and on for days and the doctor finds no signs, the health-care system often begins to fail the patient. And two of the symptoms that often appear in the total absence of clear signs of disease are fatigue and pain. These are symptoms that everyone has experienced at one time or another, usually with an appropriate cause. But when a person develops fatigue or pain nearly everywhere in her body, and the doctor can find no obvious medical cause—even if the fatigue is bone-crushing or the pain is widespread—the doctor may be inclined to dismiss the patient's symptoms as "all in her head."

Sad to say, this problem is extremely common. One study evaluated the records of 1,000 patients in an internal medicine clinic over a three-year period. Complaints of pain and fatigue producing real problems for the patient were incredibly common. Although expensive diagnostic testing was usually done, a diagnosable cause or disease was identified in only 16 percent of cases. These medically unexplained symptoms and their most serious manifestation as medically unexplained illnesses are to a large degree a problem in women's health. And medical school usually does nothing to prepare doctors to help you with this problem. If you're going to get well, you'll need to take your health into your own hands.

## The Doctor-Patient Relationship

All too often during an office visit, both patient and doctor think they're on the same page when in reality they're reading different books. For simple health problems, like a broken finger or a sore throat with a fever and swollen glands, communication between doctor and patient is usually fine. But when the patient simply does not feel "right" or is unsure of just what's bothering him or her, the doctor visit can prove unsatisfying. The reason is twofold: the way the doctor is taught to think, and changes in American society that influence how patients talk to doctors. Neither of these, of course, has anything to do with the way the patient is really feeling.

Doctor-patient relationships may be in a state of flux for a number of reasons, but the way physicians are trained hasn't changed much in recent years. So let's start with the way patients and doctors talk and listen to each other. People go to the doctor when they're unable to answer their health concerns by themselves. Since patients see doctors as experts, their relationship assumes a certain traditional, hierarchical quality: the doctor is in charge; the patient is there to listen. We can see this in the way that visits to the doctor usually proceed. The doctor controls the patient interview and rarely leaves time for the patient to voice all of his or her concerns.

While this scenario is often followed even today, education and the Internet have begun changing the doctor-patient relationship. A few years ago, a fifty-two-year-old pilot went for his annual physical exam and had his blood checked for prostate-specific antigen (PSA) levels. Although standard medical texts (and insurance companies) do not endorse using PSA as a screen for prostate cancer, it is well known that patients with prostate cancer often have elevated levels of PSA. So when the pilot's PSA rose from normal levels of 1.1 and 1.6 in prior years to 3.9, he became concerned. His doctor told him not to worry since the levels still were within normal limits, but the pilot said he wanted his prostate gland biopsied. This was done, and a tiny area of malignancy was found. When it came time to determine what to do about this cancer, the pilot was better informed than the doctor. And perhaps not surprisingly, more recent information indicates that prostate cancer is not a rare occurrence even with low levels of PSA; the pilot was right to be concerned about the change in his levels. As we all know, medical knowledge is always evolving, for doctors as well as for patients. What is fact today might not be correct tomorrow.

Such stories are not unusual in this era of easy access to medical knowledge. Even though I consider myself an expert in my field, it's not unusual for one of my patients to tell me about a new study on medically unexplained fatigue or pain about which I was unaware. Access to information and knowledge empowers the patient and often makes her more demanding of the doctor, who is bound to notice. The well-informed patient wants to be treated more as an equal rather than in the usual role of someone who asks for advice and then is expected to take it. But despite the American public's growing interest in medicine, most elements of the traditional doctor-patient relationship remain unchanged. For example, I always address my patients as Mr. or Ms. and never use their first names. Very often, a patient will ask me to use his or her first name. Many doctors will do so, but I prefer not to. I explain to my patients that I can't use their first names because I wouldn't want them to use mine. Strange as it may seem, being Dr. Natelson carries magic with it that may lead to better outcomes for my patients than we'd see if I were Benjamin to them. Later in this book, I'll explain how positive beliefs can be health enhancing while negative beliefs can make a sick person sicker.

But even when a physician makes major efforts to understand the patient's concerns, beliefs, and opinions about his or her health—and strives to communicate clearly back to the patient—it is amazing just how often doctor and patient really are not on the same page. During my own office visits, the last thing I do is to go over the plan of treatment with my patient, listening to any questions or concerns he or she may have and doing everything possible to make sure that he or she understands how we'll be proceeding. I carefully note my recommendations on the patient's chart so I can check on his or her progress at the next office visit.

But things don't always go as planned. Although people often agree to try a medicine or to see a recommended consultant, when they return to see me I'm often surprised by what they did (or did not do). Some tell me they either did not try the medicine or took it only once with horrible side effects, or decided that the consultant I suggested was just too far away for convenience. Of course, if the patient had called me, I might have been able to intervene more quickly, perhaps adjusting the dosage of the medication or explaining why a visit to the specialist was so important. But regardless, it becomes clear that a disconnect has developed despite our best attempts to communicate, and the goal at a follow-up visit is to fix this. Very often, this means less prescribing (I leave that for when we're communicating better), and a greater effort to understand how the patient copes with his or her illness.

If a patient decides not to follow my advice, I assume that he or she wasn't completely satisfied with the visit. I tell myself I must work harder to understand how the patient is feeling in order to get into agreement about how to proceed. So I encourage the patient to feel empowered and tell me at the end of our time together if we haven't covered everything that's still troubling him or her. Although this doesn't always solve the problem, it does acknowledge that there's still work to be done, that I'm trying to understand what my patient is saying, and that the patient, too, may be trying to reach a clearer understanding of my recommendations and the reasons I reached them. Doctors and patients have a lot to tell each other, especially when the patient has a clear sense of his or her symptoms but the doctor hasn't been able to identify the signs of a clearly defined disease. It's important for me to learn what the patient thinks is causing the problem. Sometimes there is a huge difference between what I think the patient is thinking and what's actually going on in his or her mind.

None of this may seem revolutionary, but it's a departure from the usual relationship between physicians and patients, where the doctor is in charge and the patient follows "doctor's orders." And, in fact, all of this flies in the face of our medical training, which teaches us to figure out the patient's chief complaint as quickly as possible, so that a diagnosis can reached. How quickly? Amazingly, one study reported that, on average, doctors listen to their patients for only eighteen seconds before jumping in and taking over the direction of the conversation. This means that patients had better know just what is bothering them, and they had better communicate it to their doctor very quickly. That's a lot to ask of the patient under any circumstance; when the patient is having a hard time describing the symptoms, it sets up an almost impossible situation for doctor and patient alike.

A number of my patients are veterans of the first Persian Gulf war, and many of them experience severe, medically unexplained fatigue. Many of these vets believe they got sick due to some exposure they experienced while on military duty, or perhaps to a vaccination they had to have for their military service. Although there is little evidence to support their beliefs, I don't tell them they are wrong, because we may never really know what triggered their illness. Being dismissive of a vet's deeply held conviction before our discussion has really gotten under way is less important than listening and setting up the groundwork for real two-way communication. So I don't worry about cause but instead focus on the symptoms themselves, remembering that the symptoms are certainly very real.

If I took the other tack and simply told the Gulf war veteran that his or her assumptions were wrong, that first visit would probably be the last. If the doctor is insensitive to the discrepancy between his or her take and that of the patient, the doctor will find the patient uncooperative and perhaps angry, and the patient will feel as if the doctor does not care or understand why he or she is there. Obviously with such a negative experience, the patient will never return. That's not what a good doctor wants to have happen.

Doctors have begun studying just how well they communicate with their patients. One study was done on 565 patients who had general medical examinations, or GMEs, at the famous Mayo Clinic in Rochester, Minnesota. Although doctors are under a great deal of pressure to reduce the amount of time they spend with patients, they usually devote up to an hour to GMEs, since they are often done on new patients or on patients who haven't visited for an extended period. The researchers studied how often the doctor and the patient agreed on the reason for the office visit. They found that agreement was high in 80 percent of the visits, but low in the remaining 20 percent. Three factors were predictive of poor agreement between patient and doctor: when the patient was a woman; when the patient had more than one reason for seeing the doctor; and when the doctor knew the patient from a previous visit. If you're reading this book, chances are you fit into one or more of these categories. You can see why finding yourself on the same page as your doctor and reaching a coherent diagnosis and treatment plan may have eluded you for so long.

## The Doctor-Patient Disconnect

During a visit, the doctor is looking for simple and straightforward explanations, but you and your problem may not fall into that category, and your physician's training may not help when the cause is unclear or you're experiencing more than one problem—for example, fatigue and pain at the same time. The kinds of problems that perplex doctors are not uncommon. Complaints like lower back pain, fatigue, dizziness, and abdominal pain are all among the top twenty-five reasons that patients set up an appointment for either an initial physician consultation or an annual checkup. How does the average doctor deal with patients whose symptoms are hard to explain?

Unfortunately not too well, and the problem is worse when the doctor is a man rather than a woman. The doctor will be aware of an extensive psychiatric literature labeling patients with unexplained symptoms as "somatizers" or "hypochondriacs." We'll discuss these labels in more detail later, but they've been around long enough to cause many generalists, family doctors, and internists to apply them in all too many cases. You see your symptoms as real; your doctor looks skeptical and makes a mental note that you're a "crock" or a complainer. Your doctor becomes dismissive, saying that he can't find anything wrong with you, that there is nothing he can do for you, or that your problem is "all in your head." He might tell you just to grin and bear it or even refer you to a psychiatrist. Certainly, he thinks there's "nothing wrong."

By dismissing you and, in essence, telling you to take care of yourself, the doctor is abrogating his job. If you're like most patients facing unexplained illness, you'll respond by becoming even more anxious to get an answer, so you'll make another appointment or decide to find another doctor. This vicious cycle often continues until you find a doctor who will listen and attend to your complaints. And what if you can't? In my experience, it is not uncommon to learn that the patient turned toward some form of alternative medicine—chiropractic, naturopathy, homeopathy, or the like—to find someone who would listen and try to help. I will share my thoughts concerning some of these alternatives with you in chapter 10.

Your original doctor not only hasn't done his job, he's risked letting things get worse by leaving you to fend for yourself. That physician either has no appreciation for how medicine progresses or for what a doctor's responsibility really is. And sadly, I see the roots of this phenomenon all the time when I try to teach these important lessons to new medical students.

Have you ever heard of dropsy? Don't be too hard on yourself if you haven't. When I make clinical rounds with fourth-year medical students—a few short months before they attain their M.D.'s—I ask them if they've ever heard this word. Only the rare student replies yes. Dropsy, in fact, is a diagnosis never made in the twenty-first century. But in the eighteenth century, dropsy was a household word. Whenever a physician saw a patient who had swelling in the feet and lower legs and whose breath gave out after minimal exertion, he would make the diagnosis of dropsy. Then, in the middle of the eighteenth century, British physicians started doing autopsies and learned that diseases in many organs could produce the same set of signs and symptoms. Although the name "dropsy" didn't disappear from medical textbooks overnight, eventually laboratory tests were developed to pinpoint the actual causes of disease in different organs. Blood tests identified kidney and liver disease, and X-rays heart disease. Patients with sick hearts that could not pump adequately often had swelling of the legs and complained of shortness of breath when they walked. What had once been labeled "dropsy" could now be attributed to congestive heart failure or some other specific disease. So dropsy became a quaint term from yesteryear. Today we know the myriad things that can lead to a failing heart: infection, coronary artery disease, toxins, and so on. The challenge for tomorrow's researchers is to understand the causative factors in order to identify an "etiologic disease entity": a definite disease with a definite cause.

Sometimes when we don't yet understand the direct cause of a certain set of symptoms, we nonetheless realize that the same symptoms repeat themselves over and over in thousands of patients. We call these identifiable sets of symptoms "syndromes." Fibromyalgia, one of the conditions we'll look at in this book, is a syndrome. Giving a name to a set of symptoms is a major step forward for two reasons: it stops the patient's search for a diagnosis while providing a framework for research, even though we don't yet know enough about its causes to make a definitive judgment (although, as we'll see later in this book, we're beginning to know a lot more). It's safe to say, though, that when no biomedical marker exists for a syndrome, doctors are sometimes too willing to attribute it to psychological factors.

A splendid example of this phenomenon is a syndrome called *torsion dystonia*. This illness, which occurs predominantly in Ashkenazic Jews, causes certain muscle groups to twist into weird-appearing shapes, causing odd, disabling movements. In the heyday of psychoanalysis, patients with torsion dystonia received hundreds of sessions of intensive psychoanalysis with no positive results. Their symptoms failed to lessen. With more intensive scrutiny, researchers learned that torsion dystonia occurred in population groups besides Ashkenazic Jews. Although no biomedical marker was ever discovered to diagnose this disorder, medical progress was finally able to identify an irregular genetic mechanism for this abnormality that was passed from parents to children.

Similarly, when I was a medical student, schizophrenia was thought to be a psychological disorder. Slowly the pendulum of medical opinion has swung to the other extreme: although there is no specific diagnostic test for schizophrenia, the illness is thought to be due to a disease of the brain, and patients with schizophrenia of long duration are known to develop evidence of chronic brain disease in the form of loss of brain tissue, or atrophy. Using advanced computer techniques, researchers at the University of Pennsylvania are developing methods to add up these defects to an actual diagnosis. Even migraine headaches are a syndrome. We don't know what causes them, although we've begun to identify more of their characteristics. But at least we've learned enough to develop drugs that can nip a migraine attack in the bud.

When medicines that don't affect psychiatric status achieve positive results in an illness, physicians can see that the symptoms are not "all in your head." Instead, physical abnormalities must be making the patient ill, without necessarily providing the concrete signs that would enable a doctor to diagnose a specific disease. So the "crock" patient is not a crock. The illness isn't made up, but really exists—just not in a form with which doctors are comfortable.

In time, the medical profession should come to understand more of these hard-to-diagnose syndromes, providing a template for medically unexplained illness: chronic fatigue syndrome (CFS), fibromyalgia (FM), irritable bowel syndrome (IBS), and others. For some people the cause may be psychological, but not for others. And regardless of what is causing these ailments, people with these symptoms will still be suffering and in need of treatment. As I will make clear throughout this book, helping patients deal with suffering is the job of the doctor.

## How Medicine Is Organized

So let's return to the doctor-patient disconnect: the idea that your physician's preconceived notions may be getting in the way of his or her ability to treat you. Unlike surgeons—who are trained to carry out specific procedures that cure people (or, at least, dramatically reverse a disease)—most physicians aren't procedure-driven but *patient*-driven. Their job is to identify and understand the problems affecting the health of their patients and then help both the patient and the patient's family cope with the problem. The number of diseases that a physician can cure remains terribly small, limited for the most part to infections, vitamin deficiencies, and the rare cancer. Thus instead of curing, the physician must be satisfied with caring, and with reducing the suffering and loss of quality of life produced by a patient's symptoms. Your job as a patient is to find a physician who understands that this is his or her job. Such a physician will not reject you because you are "difficult" or because he or she does not understand your problem.

Finding such a doctor is not simple, however. The doctor with a new MD degree may be initially idealistic and understand the nature of the job. But life intervenes. The doctor finds the demands on time to be so great that he or she can't "afford" the time to listen to patients. And those demands are only getting worse, since the medical practice is now managed by businesspeople who require delivery of more services in less time. In today's environment, even many idealistic young doctors begin to prefer "easy" patients to "difficult" ones. I've seen this unfortunate transformation in some of my younger colleagues.

Part of my practice has to do with clinical immunology, and I have tried repeatedly over the years to enlist a colleague—a talented allergist and clinical immunologist—to join me in my practice. He says, "Why would I want to do that? Your patients are really hard!" In contrast, his are easy. A twenty-eight-year-old woman with horrible hay fever comes into his office with her nose stuffed and her eyes teary. In ten minutes my friend can arrive at a diagnosis and recommend treatment. In two days, the patient is completely free of symptoms. Contrast that clinical anecdote with the forty-four-year-old woman who comes to her doctor complaining of horrible fatigue. When all the lab tests come back normal, her doctor is stuck. Yes, he can continue to do tests, but these could *all* turn out to be normal. Instead, he tries to send her on her way, even though he knows he's failed to deliver for his patient. Failure is always uncomfortable, and so it is easy to understand why this doctor might not want to see this patient again.

Remember the Mayo Clinic study we discussed earlier? What it really tells us is that "complicated" patients aren't all that unusual. Yes, 80 percent of the patients evaluated reported that they and their doctors agreed on the reasons for the office visit. But what about the remaining 20 percent? One recent medical paper concluded that a critically important task for twenty-first-century internists is to actively take on the health concerns of such patients and to be aware that in some clinics—especially those dealing with neurological and gynecological problems—caring for these complicated patients "constitutes the majority of the work." It is about them that I lecture my students. Doctors have not gone to medical school to diagnose and treat only sore throats or mild hypertension. Their own physicians' assistants can easily do this, with far less training. We doctors have learned all the material we have been taught so that we can take on difficult problems: operate on the brain tumor that looks like a killer and help the patient who has illness but not disease.

So what happens to you when you are in the doctor's office? If you find yourself speaking to a physician who either doesn't listen or cuts you off after listening for only a few seconds, you too have seen a symptom: your doctor is exhibiting what I call the three Bs—brash, boorish, and overbearing. This doctor will not be of much help to you.

Finding the appropriate doctor is often difficult, but you have the right to a physician who listens, takes you seriously, and tries to help. For whom should you look? For starters, try to find a doctor trained in family practice. These doctors are the closest to the general practitioners of yesterday. In contrast to specialists who have to be expert in a tiny part of the body, the family practitioner is a generalist and has extensive training in marrying the principles of psychiatry to those of medicine. The broad training of such doctors makes it less likely that you'll find yourself cut off in midsentence as you describe your symptoms.

Another way to reduce the chances of getting a doctor with the three Bs is to turn to a female physician. It's actually been shown that male doctors tend to be more dismissive of unexplained symptoms than female doctors. We did an early study in which patients with CFS reported feeling stigmatized by male doctors more so than by female doctors. In addition, female physicians are usually better listeners than their male colleagues. Moreover, female doctors are much less dismissive of complaints when test results come back negative. So a female family practitioner could be the best bet for someone who has symptoms for which the doctor can find no cause.

Finding a sympathetic and caring female physician, however, is partly a matter of geography. California has the highest percentage of female physicians—12 percent of the country's total. After California, there are seven states with high numbers of female physicians—New York, Texas, Illinois, Pennsylvania, Massachusetts,

Florida, and New Jersey. Female physicians in those states make up an additional 39 percent of the total for the entire country. So if you live in one of these eight states, you may have an easier time finding a female physician than you'd have in one of the other forty-two states. But with more and more women entering medical school, these numbers will improve in the near future.

I've laid out some of the reasons for doctors' inability or unwillingness to communicate not to scare you, but to show you why you need to be careful not to fall through the cracks of orthodox medicine. If you already find yourself in this situation, I hope you'll see that your frustrations *do* make sense and *shouldn't* be dismissed. Understanding the reasons why these cracks exist should empower you to find a doctor who can help you with your health problems. And understanding what modern medicine knows about these syndromes—clinical disease entities characterized by widespread pain, bone-crushing fatigue, and difficulty with attention and concentration—should help you cope better, too.

## Tips on Choosing a Doctor

A couple of things will naturally help you communicate with your doctor. If you have been seeing the same doctor for a period of time, you will have developed a relationship. That helps. The opposite of this is going to an emergency room or to an urgicare center ("doc-in-a-box"). These doctors do not have time to take care of anyone who has an illness more complicated than a sore throat or a sprained ankle. Doctors in academic centers often have surprisingly large amounts of time to devote, especially to people with complicated or hard-to-diagnose disorders. So if you have been ignored by one doctor too many, try to find a doctor in a medical school. And again, you will probably feel more comfortable with a female doctor.

## Where Do We Go Next?

Up to this point, I just wanted to set the stage and give you some answers to why you have felt so frustrated in trying to find out why you feel so lousy. The major thing I have done thus far is to give you some ground rules to help you find a doctor who does not have the three Bs. Some of you may have gotten to the end of this chapter and are thinking: "But I've looked all over for a doctor who will help me, and I've had no success." What then? Well, basically, that's the rest of this book.

In the first part of this book, I am going to show you how I take care of a patient new to my practice. First I listen, then I think about that specific patient's story. Then I do a set of diagnostic tests that I will detail for you in the next chapter. The results of that testing allow me to make a diagnosis, usually a syndrome. Just getting a diagnosis is often a relief. No more "nothing wrong." But it is not just the need for a diagnosis that drives many to keep searching; it is the relief that comes with being listened to and being understood.

Let me be clear: I don't want you to act as your own doctor, but I do want you to be informed. Furthermore, I want you to understand the best of what is available for you and your symptoms. My goal is to lay out a strategy for wellness that you can share with your doctor.

# 2

# Tests You Should Expect
# and Why

We're taught to believe that doctors have all the answers, so it often comes as an unpleasant surprise when the opposite proves to be the case. Doctors are trained to know a lot, but there is often a lot they don't know, as in cases where your doctor can't figure out the basis of your medical problem. So it's important for you to understand the way doctors deal with not knowing. In this chapter, I want to give you a good sense of what's really going on in your doctor's mind when you go to his or her office asking for help. I want you to understand how a doctor thinks after you have told him your story. This may give you a better sense of how you can present your symptoms effectively, and also of what you can and should expect from your doctor.

Almost like a detective, your doctor hunts for clues that point to a diagnosis and picks up clues from two sources:

- The story you tell about your illness: how it started, what it looks or feels like (your symptoms), what makes it better, and what makes it worse. Doctors call this information the history.
- A physical examination, organized to find bodily abnormalities or signs that point to a diagnosis.

The combination of specific *symptoms* and *signs* add up to diagnostic possibilities in the doctor's head, and he or she will then order laboratory tests in an effort to confirm the diagnosis.

When things add up, the doctor is on the case. Here's an example of how this works. Say you come into the doctor's office complaining of feeling feverish and having a bad cough. On physical examination, the doctor finds that you have a temperature of 102 degrees, and hears crackles—evidence of infection—when listening to your lungs with the stethoscope. That combination of symptoms and signs points to the diagnosis of pneumonia. To confirm this diagnostic impression, the doctor orders a chest X-ray, which will show distinct abnormalities in the lung if he or she is right.

So the symptoms you report, plus the signs the doctor finds, add up to a diagnosis. But sometimes this simple equation cannot be followed, and that's when problems arise. Let's look at another example. You'd been feeling perfectly well, when you suddenly experienced five days of horrible diarrhea, with bad nausea and a fever. Eventually the fever went away, but you're left with pain in your abdomen and diarrhea that continues to come and go. Over-the-counter medicines haven't helped much, and now you've turned to your physician.

Your doctor listens to the story of your illness and does a physical examination. Unfortunately, all the doctor can find is some tenderness in your abdomen and it's not in any specific spot, so it's not helpful in the diagnosis. He or she tests your urine and blood to check for infection, and, finding nothing wrong, orders an X-ray of your abdomen. But the X-ray doesn't turn up any problems either. Your doctor is stumped. There's only one apparent sign that something is wrong—the tenderness in your abdomen. As far as the tests are concerned, you ought to be feeling fine, which you obviously aren't.

And often, there is not even one single sign, just your symptoms. Remember Sarah Jones, the woman I described in chapter 1? That's exactly what happened in her case. She'd been feeling well and then suddenly came down with a flulike illness that simply never went away, leaving her fatigued and with a continuing sick feeling. On examination, Mrs. Jones's first doctor found nothing seriously wrong, just a slightly red throat that was too common a sign to help her solve the diagnostic equation. Because so many ill-nesses can produce fatigue and a sense of feeling ill, the doctor turned to the laboratory. With just a few tubes of blood, she was able to evaluate and then eliminate most of the medically known causes of fatigue and malaise.

Obviously, Mrs. Jones's case was going to take more investigation (and thought) to solve. Also obviously, the results of tried-and-true medical procedures and reliable tests weren't going to provide the answers she or her doctor needed. Without effective communication between Mrs. Jones and her physician, however, she might have felt almost as badly about the care she was receiving as she did physically.

Doctors don't always think to go into great detail when describing why they order certain tests and what it means when these tests fail to provide answers—information that, as it happens, proved crucial to solving Mrs. Jones's case and allaying her fears. So it's worth pausing to look at the five most common test "panels" doctors order. You're probably going to have these tests done on yourself and have perhaps taken some of them already. These panels look for alterations in blood cells, abnormalities in the function of the major organs, abnormalities in the function of the thyroid gland, evidence of some sort of infection, and rheumatological disease. Let's look at each of them briefly.

## Common Tests for the Causes of Fatigue

If you've watched medical dramas like *ER* on television, you've probably heard of the CBC, or complete blood count. This test provides information about two major causes of fatigue: alterations in the quantities of red and white blood cells. When the number of red blood cells is low, the patient is said to be *anemic* (quite common); when the red cell count is high, the patient is said to be *polycythemic* (not too common). The job of red blood cells is to carry oxygen throughout the body to allow bodily function to work normally. When the numbers of these cells decline, fatigue sets in quickly, especially after you exert yourself. If you've ever flown from a low-altitude city like New York or Los Angeles to a very high one like Denver or Salt Lake City, you may have experienced symptoms similar to anemia. With oxygen so thin in these "mile-high" cities, your normal complement of red blood cells is inadequate to supply your body with all the oxygen you need. Unless you take time to get acclimated to your new, higher altitude, with any physical exertion at all you'll quickly experience such symptoms as fatigue, insomnia, headache, and even shortness of breath. But if you stay at high altitude for a day or two, your body starts responding to the altitude stress by making more red blood cells (so much so that some people living at high altitudes have mild polycythemia). Now your organs can get the oxygen they need to keep you going at your usual pace, and your symptoms will disappear, leaving you feeling normal again.

Imagine feeling these symptoms, though, in your regular, low-altitude life, without climbing a mountain or running a marathon, and you'll have some idea of what it feels like to be anemic. A woman named Hannah Herrington came to me with exactly this problem—her red blood cell count was only about half of normal. Further tests revealed evidence of an autoimmune disorder. For unknown reasons, Mrs. Herrington's body was making substances called *antibodies* that targeted and killed her red cells. Her anemia was clearly the cause for the horrible fatigue she reported having.

Mrs. Herrington's doctor sent her to a hematologist (a blood doctor). He said that he thought she had systemic lupus erythematosis and sent her to a rheumatologist because he did not take care of patients with lupus. The rheumatologist disagreed that she had lupus but offered no further suggestions. Mrs. Herrington was still fatigued, and her red blood cell count was still too low. Even though she clearly had a serious medical problem, her doctors let her fall between the cracks, and of course Mrs. Herrington's original complaint of fatigue remained exactly the same. When she showed up at my office, I immediately understood the cause of her fatigue and realized she was in my office due to the failure of her specialists to take charge of her and her illness. So I called her family doctor and suggested that she at least treat Mrs. Herrington's symptoms until her other doctors sorted out who would do what. They gave her a blood transfusion, and the fatigue was immediately gone. The family doctor realized that the medical profession had not been doing Mrs. Herrington a service and made sure this would not happen again in the future.

In contrast to red blood cells, your white blood cells provide information about infection. When the number of these cells is high, and the person has a fever, the doctor can infer that a bacterial infection exists. When the number of these cells is low and the person has a fever, the doctor can infer that a viral infection exists. In both these conditions, feeling fatigued and sick are the most common patient complaints.

The second blood panel provides information on a number of different factors that can produce fatigue: the amount of salts in the blood (sodium, potassium, and calcium) and how the liver and the kidneys are working. When the liver fails, it cannot dispose of the bile in your bloodstream, and your eyes and eventually your skin turn yellow, or jaundiced. Jaundice is a sign of a sick liver, but less severe liver problems can make themselves evident by causing fatigue.

The third common set of blood tests evaluates how well the thyroid gland is working. The thyroid, found at the base of the neck, secretes hormones that help regulate the body's metabolism. When the gland fails, the person becomes sensitive to cold, develops easy fatigability, and experiences changes in the texture and the thickness of the skin. This condition is called *hypothyroidism*. The opposite, *hyperthyroidism*, occurs when the gland is overactive, causing the patient to feel jittery and tremulous.

The next set of tests checks for hidden infection. In the northeastern United States, where I practice, Lyme disease is a common infection that can cause fatigue, and it can progress to be a major problem when doctors don't consider it. Lyme (named for the Connecticut town where it was first discovered) comes from the bite of a tiny form of deer tick and can now be easily diagnosed by a blood test. Some people will remember having one of Lyme's telltale signs—a bull's-eye-shaped skin rash—after spending some time out of doors. But many others never notice this common sign; in relatively rare cases, they may not realize they're sick until they begin to feel tired all the time.

In fact, Lyme disease proved to be the diagnosis in the case of Sarah Jones, the patient I introduced in the last chapter. When I asked Mrs. Jones about herself, she told me she spent all of her summers on Fire Island, a narrow sandbar off the coast of New York's Long Island. Fire Island is right in the middle of the "Lyme Belt," an area of the United States that's filled with deer (and the ticks they carry) and extends from the Northeast to Michigan. Somehow her doctor had not considered Lyme in evaluating her. Once Mrs. Jones's blood test came back positive for Lyme disease, antibiotic treatment quickly cured her fatigue. If only her first doctor had thought to ask her how she spent her free time, he or she might have gotten to the bottom of Mrs. Jones's "unexplained" illness easily. Tests can do a lot, but communication is also important. One warning, though: some doctors treat patients with complaints of fatigue and achiness for Lyme, even when there is no convincing evidence the patients have that infection. High doses of antibiotics, given for long periods of time, often have dangerous side effects. I never take this course of action unless I am convinced active Lyme infection exists.

In some cases, HIV, the virus that causes AIDS, can be a cause of unexplained fatigue. Fortunately, more regular awareness and early testing for this syndrome in recent years has reduced the number of cases where fatigue shows up prior to a diagnosis. Testing for AIDS is essential except when an individual has absolutely no risk factors for becoming infected: having no sexual relations at all; being a lesbian, who is at greatly reduced risk; and having no possible exposure to blood products.

Finally, hepatitis C can produce fatigue in the absence of any signs of liver disease. Like HIV, this virus is transmitted through blood and other bodily fluids. The time between infection with the HIV virus and the development of symptoms is often quite short; in contrast, many years can go by between the time of hepatitis C infection and the onset of symptoms. Therefore, it's a good idea for your doctor to test for this infectious agent if you've recently experienced the onset of fatigue, but the test is also warranted if your problem is widespread pain instead. And the test becomes a must when blood tests for liver function are at all abnormal.

The following list lays out my approach to diagnostic testing for patients with long-duration complaints of fatigue, pain, or both.

- Blood Tests on Everyone (in alphabetic order)
    - Antinuclear antibody (ANA) and rheumatoid factor (RF)
    - C-reactive protein and erythrocyte (red blood cell) sedimentation rate (ESR)
    - Creatine phosphokinase (CPK)
    - Complete blood count with differential
    - Hepatitis C antibodies
    - HIV antibody
    - Liver function tests including SGGT, an enzyme used to diagnose liver disease
    - C6 Lyme Elisa with Western Blot if positive
    - TSH/free T4/T3 (if TSH is above the average normal value)
    - Antithyroglobulin and antithyroid peroxidase antibodies
    - Serum protein electrophoresis and immunoelectrophoresis

- Blood Tests on People with Unexplained Pain
    - Anti-extractable nuclear antigen antibodies (anti-ENAs)
    - Anti-DNA antibody
    - Sjögren's antibodies
    - Tissue plasminogen (for people with abdominal pain)

- Blood Tests on People with Fatigue and Definite Elevations in Body Temperature
    - Antibodies against Epstein-Barr early antigen; if positive, do polymerase chain reaction (PCR)
    - Antibodies against parvovirus (B-19); if positive, do PCR
    - Antibodies against cytomegalovirus; if positive, do PCR
    - Antibodies against human herpes virus 6; if positive, do PCR

- Tests on People with CFS, Excessive Sleep, and/or Objective Neuropsychological Deficit
    - Brain MRI
    - Lumbar puncture

Next, several blood tests (ANA and RF) are done to diagnose the presence of either rheumatoid arthritis (RA) or systemic lupus erythematosis (SLE). While not diagnostic, finding an elevated ESR or C-reactive protein can point to the existence of these autoimmune illnesses. These are diseases in which the body's immune system mistakenly attacks itself. They occur more often in women than in men—two and a half and six times more often, respectively. And there is an overlap between autoimmune diseases and medically unexplained fatigue or pain. Fibromyalgia (FM) occurs much more often in patients with RA or SLE than would otherwise happen by chance. And one very common autoimmune disease called *Hashimoto's thyroiditis*—an illness that attacks the thyroid—occurs nearly twice as often in women with fibromyalgia than in otherwise healthy women. The fact that Hashimoto's occurs ten times more frequently in women than in men explains why low thyroid function is much more common in women than in men. And, importantly, on rare occasions Hashimoto's can attack the brain independently of attacking the thyroid. While such an autoimmune attack is usually devastating, causing weakness on one side of the body, seizures, or even coma, milder attacks could produce fatigue and brain fog. So I add tests for thyroid autoantibodies to my panel to rule out Hashimoto's. A positive result here will lead me either to a treatment for autoimmune disease or a referral to a colleague expert in these illnesses.

Mrs. Herrington, the patient with the low red blood cell count, clearly had an autoimmune disease attacking her blood cells. In the early stage of RA and SLE, fatigue can be a primary symptom. If your primary physician suspects either of these autoimmune diseases, he or she is likely to refer you to a rheumatologist, an expert in joints and ailments involving the ligaments that attach the joints to your muscles.

The only other test I order in my initial evaluation of a patient with severe fatigue or widespread bodily pain is one that measures *creatine phosphokinase* (CPK). CPK is an enzyme involved in the normal functioning of your muscles, brain, and heart. Your CPK levels can increase when you exercise vigorously, because vigorous exercise produces some muscle damage, and this damage releases CPK. This mild muscle damage explains why your muscles ache after the first day of skiing, for example. CPK levels can also increase when your muscles are injured by an autoimmune disease called *myositis*, which can produce muscle achiness, weakness, and fatigue. I'm looking for myositis when I order this test.

Although one could do $10,000 worth of blood tests to evaluate a person for fatigue, the tests I have discussed to this point rule out its most common causes. Anemia and a poorly functioning thyroid head this list. If you complain to your doctor of pain or fatigue, he or she may or may not order all of the blood tests I have discussed to this point. But the doctor should. Getting results from *all* of these tests is the first step for me in the process of ruling out known causes of fatigue or pain.

## When the Usual Tests Are Negative

After you have had blood testing, you will return to your doctor for a follow-up appointment to go over the results. If one or more of your tests is positive (meaning that it confirmed an abnormality), your doctor should explain what the result means and how he or she intends to proceed next. If, for example, a thyroid test reveals that your thyroid gland isn't working at normal levels, your doctor will tell you the diagnosis is hypothyroidism. He or she can then start you on thyroid supplements, and your symptoms should lessen over time and then disappear.

But what if the results of all of your blood tests are negative, meaning they show that everything is "normal"? The tests we've already discussed can be used to rule out the most common diseases producing fatigue or pain. But favorable results on all of them don't mean that there's nothing wrong with you, or that your symptoms are on the verge of simply vanishing. As you now know, each of the five panels I've described here is very specific. If they are positive, they are important; if they are negative, the questions of diagnosis and cause of illness remain unanswered.

So when all of the usual tests show that everything is normal, and my patient still has fatigue or pain, I then order tests for some less common disorders that can produce these two conditions. Your doctor probably will not do these additional tests unless he or she has had a continuing education course on evaluating patients for symptoms with no obvious medical cause. (Of course, if you ask your doctor to read this chapter, he or she will be more up to date.)

## Sjögren's Syndrome or Sjögren's Disease

One of the less common diseases I look for is another rheumatological ailment, Sjögren's Syndrome, which occurs ten times more often in women than in men. The syndrome is characterized by dry eyes and dry mouth, which doctors call sicca, and these symptoms are often accompanied by severe fatigue and achiness. Some people with Sjögren's can have other serious problems throughout their bodies, much like people with SLE. These people clearly have an autoimmune disease.

The cause of sicca is usually an autoimmune attack on the body's salivary and tear-producing glands. The diagnosis of Sjögren's Disease (instead of merely Sjögren's Syndrome) is made when doctors either find antibodies circulating in the blood directed to destroying these glands or when microscopic examination of these glands following a biopsy turns up evidence of their destruction by immune cells. A biopsy of a minor salivary gland is accomplished by making a small incision in the inside of the lower lip and removing one of the many bead-sized salivary glands found just under the surface of the lip in that location. Because doctors do not often send their patients for these biopsies and because most patients with complaints of dry eyes and dry mouth do not have Sjögren's antibodies, Sjögren's Syndrome is much more commonly diagnosed than Sjögren's Disease.

Over time, I realized that many of my patients with chronic fatigue were also complaining of dry eyes and dry mouth. I wondered whether they might have Sjögren's Disease, even though their blood tests didn't show Sjögren's antibodies. So I did minor salivary gland biopsies (also known as lip biopsies) on a group of my patients who complained of severe fatigue and achiness as well as on a group of healthy comparison people. Since the bottom line for diagnosis of Sjögren's Disease is evidence of immune cell destruction of minor salivary glands, I took that as the critical end result.

The results were very important and should bolster the confidence of anyone who's ever been told that the chronic fatigue she feels was all in her head. That's because my tests showed that at least some patients who complain of chronic fatigue have clearly identifiable *physical* differences on lip biopsy from those of healthy patients. Specifically, a careful microscopic evaluation revealed that a third of my patients with chronic fatigue showed immune cell attack of some of their salivary glands. Why is this study so important? Two conclusions provide the answer: Quite a few patients with severe, medically unexplained fatigue and sicca have undiagnosed Sjögren's Disease, an autoimmune disease, as the cause of their problem. This finding plus the fact that Hashimoto's thyroiditis, another autoimmune disease, is twice as common in FM patients than in otherwise healthy people makes the point that some patients with medically unexplained fatigue and pain may have an autoimmune disease causing their symptoms despite negative blood tests for autoimmunity. A second conclusion is that fatigue is a common problem in Sjögren's Syndrome—where patients come to the doctor with the major complaint of dry eyes and mouth.

Thanks to these findings, I now always ask my patients about dry eyes or mouth. When patients report that they have to use eyedrops frequently and always need to have a drink nearby because of dry mouth, I send them to a cornea specialist who can measure tear production in the eyes (called a Schirmer's test). While dry eyes are a symptom, low tear production is a sign that allows the ophthalmologist to confirm and actually quantify the symptom. If tear production is low, I send patients for a lip biopsy. And if the biopsy is positive, I ask them to see a rheumatologist. The rheumatologist and I can then work together to help the patient feel better. This may seem like a lot to go through to get to the bottom of chronic fatigue, but it's obviously worth it. From my point of view, it is the doctor's job to walk down this path with you in order to identify any potentially treatable medical causes of your symptoms.

## Multiple Sclerosis

Another cause of fatigue is early multiple sclerosis (MS). MS is an autoimmune disease of the brain and spinal cord. Like the other autoimmune diseases, it affects women more often than men—

twice as often, in fact. Prior to the development of brain magnetic resonance imaging (the well-known test usually called an MRI), MS was diagnosed only if a person had at least two episodes of totally different neurological dysfunction separated in time from each other. The symptom in one episode might be weakness or numbness on one side of the body, while the other episode might involve an experience of double vision due to weakness in the nerves of an eye. But brain MRI has made diagnosing MS simpler. Now a doctor looks at an image that shows the brain from front to back and side to side. If someone has one attack but an MRI showing brain abnormalities that come and go over time, the diagnosis of MS will come earlier than in the past. This is important because new treatments exist for MS to greatly slow its progression.

The good news is that MS is uncommon in patients who have no complaint other than fatigue; however, over the years I have diagnosed MS in several women whose doctors had found no obvious cause for their fatigue. I image the brain of any patient whose history suggests past neurological signs; these might include weakness or numbness on one side of the body, an episode of blindness in an eye, or double vision. I also image the brain of a patient who has to sleep at least twelve hours or more a night, a condition called *hypersomnia* that suggests underlying brain disease. I'll talk more about hypersomnia later in this chapter.

## Blood Disorders

Rarely, certain malignancies of the blood can result in feelings of fatigue, even though a complete blood count shows no abnormalities. Two tests that can identify some of these malignancies are a *serum protein electrophoresis*, or SPEP, and an *immunoelectrophoresis*, or IEP. The first test provides information on the amount of blood immunoglobulins in your system; these constitute the body's antibodies. A much more common test result than the possibility of malignancy, in my experience, is the finding of minor increases or decreases in these substances in people with severe and long-lasting fatigue or pain. Sometimes deficiencies in immunoglobulins—especially in several of the components comprising immunoglobulin-G—can predispose people to repeated infections. If laboratory testing can confirm this subclass deficiency, then treatment by immunoglobulin injections may help. But this disorder is not common.

The SPEP provides the doctor information about the amount of each of the three immunoglobulins (A, G, and M) in the blood. IEP, on the other hand, provides the doctor more detail about the constitution of each of the immunoglobulins. The resulting graph shows a picture characterized by smooth increases and decreases. In rare cases, there will be a sharp spike, which is abnormal and could be a sign of multiple myeloma, a blood malignancy. When I see such a spike, I send the patient to a hematologist for further testing. Fortunately, none of my patients with these spikes has had a malignancy. The diagnosis they then receive is benign monoclonal gammopathy (BMG). BMG is not thought to produce any symptoms, but patients with this diagnosis need to be followed over time by a hematologist because some do go on to develop multiple myeloma.

About 40 percent of patients I see report that their illness started suddenly after they contracted a bad flulike viral illness. By the time I see these patients, they usually no longer have any evidence of infection. But a small percentage of patients that I care for do continue to have some evidence of infection: temperatures of over 100 degrees, abnormal white blood cell counts, or enlarged lymph nodes. You're probably familiar with these nodes even if you didn't know what they are. Usually, at the same time you experience a very bad sore throat, you'll also feel tender lumps in your neck. These are lymph nodes, and they're enlarged because, as part of your immune system, they're actively trying to respond to the throat infection. When I find objective evidence of an ongoing infection, I usually check the blood for evidence of viral infection by one of the herpes viruses.

## Herpes and Epstein-Barr Virus

Several of the herpes viruses are responsible for causing infectious mononucleosis, an illness usually seen in adolescents and characterized by a fever, a bad sore throat with swollen glands, and severe fatigue. Nearly 10 percent of people who get mono still have symptoms of "postinfectious fatigue" six months later. The relation

between bad viral infection and long-lasting illness led to the idea
that patients might have chronic mononucleosis. Because a major
cause of mono is infection with the Epstein-Barr virus (EBV), doctors inferred that EBV was the cause of chronic fatigue. So in the
1980s, doctors tested for this virus and frequently found their
patients to be positive. This result led many of them to believe that
their patients had what they called chronic Epstein-Barr infection.
Doctors began to order EBV tests in any patient with chronic
fatigue, even if they had no evidence of infection. Their line of
thinking was encouraged when the tests came back positive.

But there's a problem: just about everyone is found to be positive
for most of the tests for EBV. I am, and you probably are, too; so
are the tests of a huge number of people who are in good health.
People usually get an Epstein-Barr infection in childhood, where it
looks like one of the many viruses a kid gets. The infection is only
dramatic when an adolescent or an adult gets it. Researchers studying EBV have found that people who seemed to have "chronic
mono" actually showed similar EBV tests to perfectly healthy people for the most part. So today, the idea of chronic EBV infection
is disappearing, although I still get patients with chronic fatigue
who have been told they have chronic EBV infection. I'll have more
to say about this issue later in this chapter.

Another problem that led to confusion was the nature of the test
itself. When a foreign agent like the EB virus attacks the body, the
body responds by making antibodies to kill the virus and remove
its remains. Some of these antibodies, specifically those against the
virus's surface or capsid, remain in the body forever so their levels
can be high, even in healthy people who had the virus as children
whether they knew it or not. So testing for these antibodies isn't a
very useful way to assess a patient with chronic fatigue and prior
evidence of infection. In contrast, it does make sense to test for
antibodies against the EBV's early antigen (EA), a material
released by the virus when it is active and replicating. High antibody levels against the EBV EA does suggest a new or "reactivated" infection. Unfortunately, today most labs just tell the
doctor if the antibody level is positive or not. This is not very helpful since this test can be positive in healthy people.

I mention reactivated viruses because some viruses never go away, even after your body fights off the symptoms they produce. They merely go into hiding, a condition that virologists call "going latent." Herpes viruses are one of the best-known classes of virus that cause chronic infection. The cold sore is the most common sign of activity of one herpes virus, herpes simplex (HSV). The first infection usually occurs in childhood as a generalized viral illness with a fever, malaise, and achiness—the usual symptoms kids get. Although these symptoms quickly go away, the virus becomes latent in a branch of the nerve that carries feeling from around the mouth. Current understanding is that the body's immune system works effectively to hold the virus back from actively reproducing and causing symptoms of infection. For some but not all people, the virus can occasionally become reactivated. Then these people will develop a new cold sore. A doctor can actually culture active herpes simplex virus from one of these sores.

As you might imagine, researchers are interested in which factors make some people susceptible to repeat infections. The major factor is *immune dysregulation*, which can result from a number of causes. Stress is high among them; it makes the body act as if the immune system were working on only two cylinders. With the system compromised, the virus can become active again, and the patient may experience a new cold sore. With a disease like AIDS, where the immune system is partially destroyed, cold sores are often a major problem.

AIDS patients can become quite sick with reactivated EBV. And rarely, patients without AIDS can actually develop chronic active EBV infection. In all of these patients, active virus can usually be found, and antibodies against early antigen can be found at high levels. In contrast to people with chronic fatigue, these patients are usually extremely sick, with evidence of disease in the liver, lungs, or eyes. It's important to know that people with chronic fatigue *rarely* have very elevated levels of antibodies against early antigen—results that would, indeed, suggest chronic EBV infection. And, in my experience, even if that test is inconclusive, a more sensitive test that looks for the virus itself (known as the polymerase chain reaction, or PCR), rather than for antibodies reacting to its presence, has never been positive. With low levels of antibodies against early antigen and negative PCR testing for EBV, our current understanding is that people with chronic fatigue don't have reactivated EBV.

However, Ron Glaser, a virologist at Ohio State University, has come up with a neat idea to explain how EBV infection could lead to chronic fatigue even in the absence of the complete virus itself. In some situations, the virus starts replicating, but the body's immune system tamps down this process by attacking viral subcomponents. Glaser hypothesized that these subcomponents themselves could produce symptoms. He tested this by injecting mice with the EBV early antigen, which is not infectious. Nevertheless, the injection produced a dramatic decrease in the activity levels of the mice for up to two weeks, an effect Glaser interpreted as fatigue. His line of thinking is that some people might be sensitive to toxic effects of viral EA, which could be released even if the body can stop total replication of the virus. There is a long distance between mice and humans, but this is an interesting idea.

A number of other herpes viruses can cause infectious mononucleosis, and, using the same train of logic as with EBV, these viruses have been implicated in causing chronic fatigue and widespread pain. These include cytomegalovirus (CMV), human herpes virus 6 (HHV-6), and human herpes virus 7 (HHV-7). Several research reports implicate the last two of these herpes viruses in producing chronic fatigue, but no clinical test is available to doctors in practice to confirm this possibility. So as of now, these other herpes viruses are in the same league as EBV.

## TB and Chlamydia Pneumoniae

In completing my evaluation of patients with fatigue and a low-grade fever, I check to be sure their doctor has done a skin test to rule out tuberculosis (TB). Although not common in middle-class America, TB is still around and in some cases produces no symptoms other than fatigue. I then finish up by testing for antibodies against two other infectious agents. The first of these is parvovirus B19. Although usually a disease of children, this infectious agent can produce a flulike illness in adults, characterized by a skin rash, fatigue, and joint achiness. Even if there is no history of a rash, I test for this virus when there is a hint of infection. The second infectious agent is chlamydia pneumoniae, a common cause of respiratory infection and one that is implicated in some cases of chronic fatigue (the other chlamydia you may have heard of as a sexually transmitted disease is a different strain of the same bacteria). If testing is positive, both of these agents can be treated by an infectious diseases specialist.

## Chronic Sinusitis

Some people with chronic fatigue or widespread pain will mention that they also have other recurring symptoms, or their past medical record may make note of such conditions. For example, it's not uncommon for a chronic fatigue patient to report having had repeated attacks of sinusitis. When this is the case, I ask the patient if he or she has problems with stuffed nose, postnasal drip, and pain or pressure in the face. Answering yes suggests the existence of chronic sinusitis, and then I try to confirm that diagnosis by doing a CT scan of the sinuses, which are located just under and above the eyes. The scan can reveal radiographic evidence of chronic sinus infection, usually seen as a thickening of the sinus linings. A chronic infection of this kind, as is the case with so many infections, can produce chronic fatigue and many of the ancillary symptoms. When evidence for chronic sinusitis is found, I refer the patient to an ear, nose, and throat specialist for treatment.

# After Testing Is Completed

We've just spoken of a large number of tests, some involving the blood, others involving MRIs and other kinds of scans. It would be tempting to think that after such a detailed workup, your physician will likely find an underlying cause for your chronic fatigue or pain. While this may be the case for some patients, it certainly is not for many who wind up in my office. The result of this extensive workup for infectious agents is nearly always negative. So the chances of finding evidence of ongoing infection in someone with chronic infectious-type symptoms is, in fact, rare. Why do I order so many tests? Well, in a relatively small number of patients, one or more of these tests may, in fact, reveal an infection or other medical cause that is treatable. And, of course, there's no way to rule out an infectious agent without testing for it. If this detailed workup proves negative, there are still other kinds of tests to carry out. We'll simply know that an infection is likely not the root of your problem.

## Beyond Infection: Neuropsychological Testing

Many of the patients who consult with me complain of "brain fog." They say they forget things, get lost while driving, and have difficulty concentrating. They report that their problem gets worse if they are in a noisy environment or one with other distractions. We've done *neuropsychological testing* on these patients, and our own research has proven that some patients with these complaints do show abnormalities. They feel they're having trouble concentrating because they are having trouble concentrating, as well as paying attention and doing complex tasks that require attention.

Neuropsychological testing is a way to assess objectively an individual's higher-order brain functions: intelligence, memory, and ability to concentrate. It can relieve the patient of fears that he or she has a progressive brain disease like Alzheimer's. Importantly, patients with brain fog rarely have problems with intelligence and with the ability to memorize; in contrast, these are the major issues in Alzheimer's.

So neuropsychological testing is a useful tool to assess the complaint of brain fog. In our work on chronic fatigue syndrome (CFS), we have found patients to have problems processing complex information. Finding such a problem can be useful in substantiating insurance or disability claims. In fact, because patients are often aware of this, some do not try to do their best on the tests. This leads to real problems because the neuropsychologist has ways to measure mental effort objectively and because the insurance companies reject disability claims for any patients who make less than a full effort on the tests.

Individuals considering testing need to be aware of two issues:

it is extensive and expensive. The neuropsychologist has to test across all cognitive functions and cannot limit the assessment just to evaluating attention and concentration. The tests themselves may take up to eight hours, and it will take the neuropsychologist nearly as long to score and interpret them, prepare a report, and then meet with you to explain the findings. As a result, testing is likely to cost between $2,500 and $5,000, depending on where you live.

Despite these costs, I find abnormal neuropsychological test results very important in determining whether any further evaluation is necessary. Abnormalities in cognitive function support underlying brain dysfunction. So when neuropsychological tests are abnormal, I do brain MRI imaging if this has not been done before in the past year. When a patient sleeps a lot, this hypersomnia also supports the idea of an underlying brain problem. While innumerable things can disturb sleep, the number of reasons why an individual sleeps for more than ten or eleven hours a night is relatively few; brain dysfunction is high on the list.

When a patient has two or three of the factors suggesting brain dysfunction—abnormal MRI, hypersomnia, abnormalities in cognitive testing—I will evaluate the spinal fluid by a procedure known as a spinal tap or lumbar puncture. Whenever I mention this procedure, patients get nervous. But in actuality the tap is less painful than getting a shot in the buttocks (though there is a risk of developing a bad headache afterward).

Why do it at all? In rare circumstances, an individual can have herpes viral infection, not in the blood but in the brain and in the spinal fluid that bathes it. So I send the fluid for routine tests, for tests looking for markers suggestive of MS, and for PCR testing looking for herpes viruses. If the fluid is positive, I send the patient to an expert in infectious diseases for treatment.

## The Workup for Irritable Bowel

Just as your doctor will order a series of tests looking for the causes of chronic fatigue or pain, he or she will also order tests if you've been diagnosed with irritable bowel syndrome (IBS). Although the diagnosis of IBS is based on symptoms, your doctor will probably want to rule out serious gut diseases that can produce similar symptoms. The most serious of these are called inflammatory bowel diseases and are diagnosed by several procedures: an X-ray study of the lower bowel (this is called a barium enema) and a biopsy of the intestinal wall during colonoscopy. This last procedure is often done under sedation, because the doctor needs to pump air into the bowel in order to see inside it, and this can be uncomfortable. Ulcerative colitis is an example of an inflammatory bowel disease, and it is often serious, making people quite ill. Although they sound similar, this group of diseases shouldn't be (and usually isn't) confused with IBS.

One illness that can mimic IBS is called gluten enteropathy, or *celiac disease*. This is a genetically related autoimmune disease in which your gut becomes allergic to wheat products and cannot absorb food materials normally. In its worst form, celiac disease can produce weight loss with resulting malnutrition, vitamin deficiencies, and diarrhea. But occasionally none of these symptoms exist, and people may instead have fatigue, achy joints, or symptoms suggestive of IBS. The initial evaluation for this disorder uses a blood test that looks for antibodies against elements within the gut. If these tests are positive, your doctor will send you to a gastroenterologist who will want to visualize and biopsy your small intestine. To do this, he or she will pass a scope, a half inch in diameter, through your mouth and your stomach, and into your small intestine. Usually this procedure is done under sedation.

One food sensitivity—lactose intolerance—is known to produce symptoms identical to IBS. In this disorder, your bowel lacks enough of the chemicals that break down the sugar lactose, which is found in milk products. A test will allow your doctor to diagnose this insufficiency. Incidentally, many people have experienced an isolated episode of food-related IBS after eating several handfuls of sugar-free candy quickly. Aspartame, the chemical with the brand name NutraSweet that is found in many candies and sodas, is non-nutritional and is not absorbed into your body. But the bacteria in your gut will attempt to treat aspartame the same way they treat lactose, and the sudden introduction of large amounts of the artificial sweetener into your system will produce huge amounts of methane gas. You'll begin to experience a bout of severe crampy pain, gas, and horrible diarrhea. Fortunately, it will go away.

## When Everything Comes Up Normal

The battery of tests and scans covered in this chapter takes many words to describe, but most of them can be done in one or two office visits. In my practice, these tests are nearly always negative, meaning that everything the tests can investigate is normal. The most common abnormalities are in the complete blood count, with some evidence for anemia, or in the thyroid tests. When I find these abnormalities, I send the patient back to his or her general practitioner to have these problems corrected. If the fatigue and pain continue despite adequate treatment of these problems, the patient returns to me. Rarely, I find evidence for an autoimmune disease such as lupus or MS.

So when the test results are all normal, what happens next? My patient's pain and fatigue are very real, and test results, whether positive or negative, won't make these sensations go away. My next steps as a doctor are therefore exactly the same as they'd be if my patient had complained about a sore throat or a broken bone. First, I briefly review with the patient the reasons for the tests we've done and their results. Then, despite the negative tests, I roll up my sleeves and use the syndromic method to make a diagnosis, and I begin to develop avenues of treatment. My patient deserves no less, even if—maybe even *especially* if—the complaints aren't easily explained. In getting to a proper diagnosis and bringing someone back to health, communication is always my number-one priority. It's frustrating, for a doctor as well as for a patient, when the underlying causes of disease remain a mystery. But at least my patient can take heart that this battery of tests has ruled out a large number of illnesses, some relatively minor and some potentially very serious.

Unfortunately, many doctors are uncomfortable with medical complaints that can't be backed up by abnormal test results.

When out of their comfort zone they may leap to the conclusion that there is nothing wrong. Whether they state this to the patient directly or merely hint at it, the effect is nearly always the same: the person feels misunderstood, ignored, or disbelieved, and more pessimistic than ever about regaining health.

I have a real problem with this trend to depend on what I call "medical materialism." That's the term I use to define the doctor's need to hold an abnormal test result in his or her hands. And when that result is not there, the doctor assumes that what the person describes doesn't exist. How unfortunate! Getting to a diagnosis despite negative test results may be difficult, but it's not impossible. Hearing the "nothing wrong" diagnosis makes you feel worse; this is the opposite of what your doctor's goal should be. So let's move on to the next step: diagnosis.

# 3

# What Doctors Know about
# Medically Unexplained Illnesses

When medical materialism works, of course, it is fabulously helpful. Medical school teaches students how diseases start and progress, and what markers they leave behind. These markers are the basis of the lab tests doctors order, and researchers work constantly to develop new markers for human diseases. But there are many examples of diseases for which the medical materialism model fails.

## The Unexplained and Somatization Disorder

Let's look at one of these diseases, because it teaches us a great lesson. Remember torsion dystonia from chapter 1. It is a neurological disorder usually found in a previously well child or adolescent of Eastern European Jewish descent. For no apparent reason, the young person develops a muscle contraction that forces his or her body into abnormal, sometimes painful, movements or postures. The disorder may start with a problem in one limb while the child is walking.

Imagine this happening in the 1950s, when medical diagnostic testing was quite primitive. The doctor does a careful examination and finds nothing unusual. Lab testing reveals no abnormalities. The adolescent patient reports that the problem gets worse with stress. Since it's the 1950s, Freudian thinking has recently swept the United States. The patient is the child of a hardworking, upwardly mobile Jewish couple. The doctor meets with the family and tells them there is nothing wrong with their child—that it is all in his or her head. Psychoanalysis begins, and the child becomes more and more physically twisted. Since the problem is not psychological, nothing results, and eventually the child becomes wheelchair bound.

As I discussed earlier, torsion dystonia was a "nothing wrong" syndrome in the 1950s. Since that time, however, medical science has advanced and identified a specific genetic abnormality that codes for muscle torsion dystonia. So torsion dystonia has gone from a mental ailment—one that doctors were sure was all in the person's head—to a genetic disorder that is definitively explained by a physical abnormality. Unfortunately, the medical profession is slow to learn from its own experience, and so the story of torsion dystonia has to be relearned over and over again.

Medicine ultimately moves forward when researchers can agree on a clinical case definition for a syndrome, one that's so far been defined only by symptoms, with no biomedical marker that can confirm the real cause. As this short history of torsion dystonia shows, the marker may be found many years later, but that doesn't make the symptoms less real in the meantime.

Medical materialism fails for every psychiatric disease in the books, from autism to schizophrenia to depression. The doctor can diagnose these diseases only by observing behavior, talking with the patient, and asking questions. The model fails for migraines, too. Migraines are another case where lab tests are useless; instead, patients must endure severe pulsing pain over half the head, accompanied by sensitivity to bright light and nausea or vomiting. But at least a definition of migraine exists, and when the symptoms add up to the clinical syndrome we call migraine, your doctor can make a diagnosis. So, too, for autism, schizophrenia, and depression. The general rule is that medical materialism fails when no lab test exists to serve as a marker of a specific disease.

Let's look at another example that illustrates how symptoms may be used to define a syndrome, even if a biomedical marker hasn't been found yet. An excellent example exists in the field of psychiatry. Back in the early 1960s, schizophrenia was diagnosed four times more often in the United States than in England. Obviously, it's possible that schizophrenia was a lot more common in the United States than in the United Kingdom. But a more probable explanation was that without a diagnostic test to help, doctors in the two countries diagnosed the illness differently. This striking discrepancy was the reason a number of psychiatrists decided to arrive at clinical case definitions for each of the many psychiatric syndromes. That effort at coding psychiatric illnesses was called the *Diagnostic and Statistical Manual of Mental Disorders* (DSM). Essentially they took the syndromic approach by diagnosing diseases based on the existence of certain symptoms. Over the years, the *DSM* has gone through four updates, with a fifth in the works. Although psychiatrists fiercely argue among themselves about certain diagnoses in the *DSM*, for better or worse it has put all psychiatrists on the same page. Schizophrenia for one psychiatrist is pretty much schizophrenia for every other psychiatrist. And having a clinical case definition with which everyone agrees allows individual doctors and researchers to pool information with other doctors and researchers. So, as you might expect, rates of schizophrenia were no different in the United States and England.

You would think that having standard definitions like these would also be helpful in the case of medically unexplained illness. But there's a big problem: the psychiatrists involved in developing clinical case definitions for psychiatric disease included medically unexplained illnesses and came up with a single definition to cover all of them, and the history of this diagnosis—called *somatization disorder*—smacks of sexism. You need to know about this diagnosis, because its existence—especially if you're a woman—may be directly responsible for doctors saying there is nothing wrong with you. Helping you cope with this disconnect between what is actually known and what has simply become medical habit is a major reason for my writing this book.

Somatization disorder (SD) is a psychiatric diagnosis usually applied to women who seek medical care for a host of physical complaints, starting before the age of thirty. A psychiatrist whose thirty-two-year-old female patient reports having had many years of bad headaches, stomachaches, frequent flu infections, and a feeling of lightheadedness would probably make the diagnosis of SD. In fact, this woman's symptoms would fulfill the official definition for SD. As far as the *DSM* is concerned, this set of symptoms—either overattention to one's bodily sensations or a set of health concerns that have no medical cause—amounts to a chronic form of worrying: in short, a psychiatric disorder. This is quite a collection of symptoms, of course, and it's not especially easy to find people exhibiting them in the American population as a whole; it describes only 0.23 percent of all women and 0.02 percent of men. But the rates are tenfold higher for patients in primary care.

One problem with the diagnosis of SD is that it attributes a psychiatric cause to medically unexplained symptoms; it ignores past examples, like torsion dystonia, where medicine made the wrong assumptions about the cause of disease, and where the physical (not psychiatric) cause was very real. But an even bigger problem with the existence of SD is that it makes doctors comfortable in saying the patient has nothing wrong, or at most a problem that is all in the head. The first problem has to do with the diagnosis itself, which lies in the opinion of the examiner.

For someone to be given the diagnosis of SD, the physician or the psychiatrist has to decide whether the symptom has a medical explanation. If everyone making such a decision answered yes to this question, then only 3 percent of patients with chronic fatigue syndrome (CFS) would receive the diagnosis of SD. But if these same physicians and psychiatrists happened to conclude that CFS symptoms had no medical explanation and were due to psychological factors, then 97 percent of patients would receive the diagnosis of SD. Now, all of a sudden, a treatable physical illness will be dismissed as "nothing wrong," and you may be told just to "tough it out."

Since the doctor's opinion determines whether he or she diagnoses patients with this disorder, what can the diagnosis mean? I do see a rare patient who is a chronic worrier and has had lifelong health concerns. Such a person may well have a psychiatric disorder. But in someone who was fine one day and sick the next, it doesn't make sense to invoke the diagnosis of SD, regardless of age.

Furthermore, once the SD diagnosis is made, the patient is often blamed for being ill. Take this story, for example. One of my patients was sent for neuropsychological testing related to a disability claim. The testing showed the expected problems that I reviewed in the last chapter. Despite this, the neuropsychologist made a diagnosis of SD and blamed the patient, claiming she had "basic ingrained personality problems." Wow! My poor patient didn't stand a chance. Not only was there nothing wrong, but the psychologist was saying that her personality forced her to make up her complaints.

You are probably asking, "Where did this thing come from?" The nineteenth century, in fact. Somatization disorder is simply a polite, more modern way to describe what used to be called *hysteria*, a term that nineteenth-century male doctors originally applied to female patients who exhibited bizarre movements (such as bending backward to make an inverse letter C). It took more than two hundred years for doctors to realize that men could have this problem too, albeit substantially less often.

Thanks to this long-held idea of hysteria, doctors were able to imagine that a disease like torsion dystonia (or any other disease with no obvious medical explanation, for that matter) derived from a family tendency toward hysteria rather than from a genetic cause. These dramatic examples of psychiatrically based symptoms became rather rare except in exceptionally stressful conditions like the battlefield. Finding a soldier who claimed he could not walk but who had an otherwise normal neurological examination led to the conclusion that such problems had no organic medical or neurological cause. Instead, they were thought to be functional, the psychological consequences of emotion-laden or highly stressful situations. In contrast to organic causes in which actual disease of the brain could be seen upon gross and microscopic examination, here the idea was that the problem was psychogenic, reflecting a more personal and individualistic reaction to stress.

What happened over time, however, was what I call definition drift. When bizarre movements and tics disappeared, as well as examples of hysterical paralysis, psychiatrists shifted their attention to people who reported multiple *other* medical symptoms that had no apparent medical cause. It was only a short leap for psychiatrists to believe that patients with such problems were also hysterical. That leap was not a logical one, however; it merely heaped new illnesses onto an old definition and had no scientific basis in fact. Among these illnesses were chronic fatigue syndrome and fibromyalgia (FM). The existence of the old idea of hysteria enabled many doctors to conclude that the illnesses didn't *really* exist. Or, more precisely, even if doctors allowed that CFS and FM existed, they could still argue that these were not diseases in and of themselves. Instead, they were functional disorders related to hysteria: they were all in the patient's head.

Over the years, the idea that these disorders were manifestations of hysteria waned and was replaced by the concept of somatization. But practicing physicians didn't miss the connection between hysteria and somatization—in the end, only the terminology had changed. It was one step from their viewing patients with chronic fatigue or widespread pain, like their Victorian predecessors, as a waste of time.

This story explains one reason for the disconnect in communication between patients and doctors when facing unexplained illnesses. Patients reported real symptoms; doctors resorted to the SD diagnosis for reasons that seemed perfectly logical to them but that made no sense to their suffering patients. Instead of medicine being based on fact, this line of thinking is based on opinion without any scientific support. That's not how medicine is supposed to work and is not the kind of "science" that has allowed so many medical advancements over the years.

The fact that the definition of somatization is circular and not amenable to scientific testing just leaves me cold. When doctors label medically unexplained symptoms as "functional somatic syndromes," they are really saying that the patient's complaints must be psychogenic, whether they tell the patient this or not. A physician who identifies you as having a "functional" problem may believe (and actually tell you) that that there's nothing wrong with you except for your magnifying or exaggerating your problem. This is just a short step away from calling your problem imaginary, an all-too-common belief among doctors. Fortunately, the pendulum seems ready to swing in the other direction. A recent editorial in the *British Journal of Psychiatry*, a major journal in its field, calls for abolishing the SD diagnosis and using a term such as "medically unexplained illness" instead. But we'll see how long it takes doctors to come around to this view.

Rather than calling medically unexplained symptoms "nothing wrong," a more rational approach has been to try to come up with clinical case definitions of these disorders; that way, researchers can identify groups of patients to study and apply scientific reasoning (not just opinion) to solve their cases. Being able to identify a group of patients based on symptoms allows doctors to establish clear-cut boundaries between that group and patients who show similar, but different, sets of symptoms. This is a research strategy that lets the researcher determine whether the illnesses are the same or different. Doing this is step number one in identifying the causes of illness.

## Severe Fatigue

So let's consider these symptoms one by one, starting with the problem of severe and long-lasting fatigue. And let's keep in mind that, as with any personal characteristic, different people may think of fatigue in different ways. In the course of my practice, I have seen a handful of women who reported that they have *always* felt tired and *always* needed to rest or nap during the day; some have even told me they suspect this is the reason that back in school they were always chosen last for sports. Many more, of course, have sought care because fatigue is a new and unfamiliar feeling to them. As with any other human property—from height to intelligence to aspects of self-image—people run along a continuum. Some are on the low side, others right in the middle, and the rest are on the high side. It's the same for fatigue. Some women may not count this as a trait while others, like some of my patients, may say it is an integral part of the way they think about themselves.

In evaluating fatigue, your doctor really should start by asking you two questions: "Is your feeling of fatigue new?" and "Does your fatigue persist even after you rest?" If you have had a problem with fatigue all your life, we can't say you have chronic fatigue syndrome; instead, you have what I call constitutional fatigue. Regardless of what we call it, we will deal with it in the next two chapters, so don't give up.

So this leaves us with those of you who have a new onset of fatigue. Fatigue is so common in everyday life that doctors don't pay attention to it unless it is prolonged, lasting at least one month. If it lasts for more than six months, it is called *chronic fatigue*. For an individual with fatigue lasting more than six months to fall within the category of having *chronic fatigue syndrome* or its less severe version, *idiopathic chronic fatigue*, the case definition says that the fatigue must be severe enough to have a major impact on that person's life. When the first clinical case definition for CFS was developed in 1988, a patient had to report that fatigue produced at least a 50 percent decrease in activity. Obviously this decrease can vary greatly from person to person, with many reporting having to cut back on activities such as going to the gym. However, an occasional patient can still jog several times a week, but reports that this is very little activity compared to previous ability.

Requiring patients to report a percentage drop in activity—whether 40 percent, 50 percent, or something else—didn't make sense. How could anyone be expected to arrive at such a number? This problem led to a revision of the case definition in 1994. Thereafter, the patient's fatigue had to produce a *substantial* decrease in personal, social, job, or school-related activities. The new case definition did not provide a guideline, however, on how this "substantial decrease in activity" was to be determined. When I speak with patients whose fatigue has lasted many months or years, I ask them to tell me how their fatigue has altered their lives, and whether their fatigue has produced a mild, moderate, substantial, severe, or very severe reduction in their activity for each of these four areas of life. By putting the word *substantial* within a range of responses, a person can do a better job of deciding where he or she fits. If a patient reports a *substantial* decrease in activity in at least one of these spheres, I ask for specifics on exactly what activities he or she no longer can do. That puts me on the same page as the patient.

So diagnosing CFS requires the doctor to communicate with the patient to determine how active he or she was prior to becoming ill, and many patients report having been very active prior to getting sick. As I mentioned earlier, someone who can still jog can have CFS. If that person previously was able to run miles every day and now can only jog around the block a few times a week, her activity level has fallen profoundly. Perhaps jogging is the only normal activity the person can carry on, other than her job. In such cases, the remainder of the patient's social or personal life may be ruined, because of the need to rest the second she returns home from work. Having had to curtail activity substantially from what it had been, that patient would fulfill the revised 1994 criterion for CFS. There's been some fine-tuning of the case definition since 1994, especially by researchers from the Centers for Disease Control, but the basic framework for diagnosis remains the same.

## Fatigue Plus Is Chronic Fatigue Syndrome

For some individuals, severe and long-lasting fatigue is the only problem. Patients with fatigue alone receive the diagnosis of idiopathic chronic fatigue. But others get what I call fatigue plus. They have fatigue *and* other bodily complaints. Only an individual in the fatigue plus category can get the diagnosis of CFS. The table on page 54 lists the additional eight symptoms used in establishing the diagnosis as well as muscle weakness and feeling feverish, from the more demanding 1988 case definition. People with CFS have at least four of these symptoms, which must have either existed or recurred during at least six consecutive months. However, the complaint of problems with memory or concentration is treated differently from the other seven symptoms. For this symptom to be counted, the person must report that it is severe enough to produce a substantial reduction from previous levels of occupational, educational, social, or personal activities.

The table contains information from patients fulfilling the 1994 case definition for CFS. Patients who reported cognitive difficulties or unrefreshing sleep tended also to have most of the other symptoms on the list. Looked at another way, those severely fatigued

## CFS-Related Symptoms and the Percentage of Other Problems with Any Single Symptom

| | Feverishness | Glands | Sore Throat | Headache | Myalgia | Muscle Weakness | Arthralgia | Exercise | Sleep | Cognition |
|---|---|---|---|---|---|---|---|---|---|---|
| Feverishness[a] | — | | | | | | | | | |
| Glands[b] | 69 | — | | | | | | | | |
| Sore Throat | 75 | 88 | — | | | | | | | |
| Headache | 75 | 75 | 85 | — | | | | | | |
| Myalgia[c] | 80 | 79 | 87 | 92 | — | | | | | |
| Muscle Weakness[a] | 76 | 75 | 84 | 87 | 93 | — | | | | |
| Arthralgia[c] | 74 | 71 | 81 | 84 | 88 | 87 | — | | | |
| Exercise[d] | 81 | 80 | 88 | 92 | 98 | 94 | 88 | — | | |
| Sleep | 81 | 80 | 87 | 92 | 98 | 93 | 88 | 98 | — | |
| Cognition | 80 | 80 | 87 | 91 | 97 | 92 | 87 | 98 | 97 | — |

[a] Symptoms no longer counted in the revised 1994 case definition to diagnose CFS.
[b] In the neck or groin or under the arms.
[c] Achy muscles and joints respectively.
[d] Complaint that even minimal exertion produces dramatic worsening of fatigue.

people who also reported a prominent sore throat had the lowest rates of other symptoms, with tender lymph glands and feeling feverish close behind. So the table tells us that if you have very bad fatigue plus cognitive problems—or fatigue plus unrefreshing sleep—you stand a very good chance of experiencing a lot of other symptoms, too. On the other hand, if you have fatigue and infectious-type symptoms (a sore throat, feverishness, or tender lymph glands in the neck, groin, or armpit), you may have relatively few other symptoms.

Another group of researchers looked at symptom frequency in CFS patients and found a fifty-fifty split between those with many and those with relatively fewer symptoms. However—and this is very significant—the "severe" symptom group was made up entirely of women. In fact, 71 percent of the women and *none* of the men fell into the severe category.

But when do you count a symptom? If you have mild problems with three of the symptoms on the list and a moderate problem with headaches, for example, do you have CFS? I would not make this diagnosis, because these symptoms are very common in otherwise well people, too. Many people have mild or even moderate problems with headaches or backaches. These symptoms are certainly real, but they may not add up to your getting the diagnosis of CFS. I never could understand why the group defining CFS required that cognitive problems had to produce a substantial problem in order to count while others did not. So I believe that to count, the symptoms should be a substantial problem for you.

If a patient reports symptoms consistent with fatigue plus, the doctor's working diagnosis is "CFS-like illness." But the doctor won't be ready to share these thoughts with you yet because the current case definition for CFS requires it to have no medical explanation. So now your physician must try to rule out medical causes for your fatigue, at least in part by ordering the initial set of blood tests we discussed in chapter 2. Finding a medical cause for fatigue means the patient does not have CFS but opens the door for medical treatment of the underlying cause. The diagnosis of CFS is also not made if a person has a serious psychiatric disease, such as substance or alcohol abuse, schizophrenia, or manic-depressive disorder. When patients with these disorders experience fatigue, it is usually thought to relate to their psychiatric problems.

CFS-like illness is fairly common, occurring in over 4 percent of the population. But after excluding medical and psychiatric causes of severe fatigue in people who may or may not have gone to the doctor for their problems, the resulting numbers with clear CFS get quite small—5 of every 1,000 women and 3 of every 1,000 men. CFS is not a common ailment. It does occur in people of Latin heritage twice as often as in African Americans or in Caucasians, and twice as often in skilled workers as in professionals. And remember, I said that the fatigue could produce a substantial decrease in school-related activities. That's the case because CFS is not limited to adults; children and adolescents can also develop this problem, albeit less often than adults. These younger patients, however, are not the focus of this book.

At this point, you may be saying to yourself, "CFS sounds as if it is my problem, but my fatigue is not that bad," or "I have bad fatigue, but I don't have all those other problems." What happens then? Do you fall between the cracks? The answer is no. You have a milder version of CFS called idiopathic chronic fatigue (ICF). Getting the diagnosis of ICF means one of two things: either your fatigue produces less than a substantial decrease in activity, or you have substantial problems with fewer than four of the symptoms on the list. Rates of ICF are about double those of CFS (about 1 percent of the population); curiously, however, I rarely see patients whose symptoms add up to this diagnosis. I'm not sure why this is the case. Either their doctors are taking adequate care of them, or, more probably, their doctors have told them there is nothing wrong and they are going it on their own.

One semantic issue that returns again and again has to do with the similarity of CFS to depression. We'll talk about this in more detail in chapter 5, but it's also relevant here. Although we usually think of depressed people as being sad or less interested in doing things they used to enjoy, truly depressed people also have somatic complaints. And there is quite a bit of overlap between those symptoms and those reported by patients who have been diagnosed with CFS but have *no* depression. These symptoms include fatigue, achiness, poor sleep, and difficulty concentrating.

Two things about CFS set it aside from depression. The first has to do with one of the key complaints of patients with CFS: that even minimal exertion makes the patient's entire set of symptoms, from fatigue to malaise, get worse. This symptom is not uncommon when fatigue is caused by a medical illness such as heart failure or anemia, but it is much less common in fatigue associated with psychiatric illness such as depression. Therefore, doctors find the "minimal exertion" symptom useful in separating fatigue in depression from fatigue in CFS.

The second difference between depression and CFS has to do with illness onset. In a telephone survey study conducted to identify CFS patients who don't necessarily go to the doctor, about 20 percent reported that they were fine one day and horribly sick the next, with something like the flu from which they never recovered. People who come to see me as patients report this sudden, flulike onset of illness at twice these rates.

When a doctor hears that an illness begins suddenly, he or she thinks of either infection or some kind of poisoning. Since poisoning is uncommon, this sudden onset of severe fatigue points to an infectious trigger. Rates of CFS approach 9 percent of patients who are initially diagnosed by blood tests as having infectious mononucleosis. And mono isn't the only infection that seems to be implicated in the onset of CFS. Some patients who have positive blood tests for Lyme disease go on to CFS. In fact, researchers have learned that just getting a bad viral illness is enough to raise the risk of developing CFS more than twenty-fold. Doctors finally seem to be learning this lesson, too. When researchers used telephone polling methods to identify patients with CFS, those who reported a sudden illness onset were much more likely to have received the diagnosis of CFS than those with a gradual illness onset (41 percent versus 6 percent).

As soon as people learn about these facts, they immediately jump to the conclusion that CFS is some sort of chronic infection. But, as I said in chapter 2, there's really no evidence for that belief. Instead, infection seems to be a *trigger* for chronic fatigue, which may sound the same but is different.

The graph below shows the dates when patients reported that they experienced a sudden onset of their illness. As you can see, the distribution isn't random. CFS begins much more often in the winter—the peak time for viral illness—than in the other seasons. This graph supports the idea that infection can trigger chronic fatigue, but, once again, data do not exist to support the idea that infection continues.

The take-home point is that getting a bad infection increases the risk for developing chronic fatigue. Interestingly, if an individual has a problem with fatigue prior to infection, that increases the risk of winding up with chronic fatigue afterward. In fact, CFS patients are more likely to report that they had experienced infectious-type symptoms and fatigue many months before the onset of their illness than other patients where fatigue is a problem, such as those with multiple sclerosis.

Another risk factor for developing problems with fatigue later in life is low blood pressure. Normal systolic pressure is 120; the break-point for systolic hypertension (what we usually call "high blood pressure") is 140; and systolic hypotension (low blood pressure) is defined as a pressure less than 100 mmHg. In one

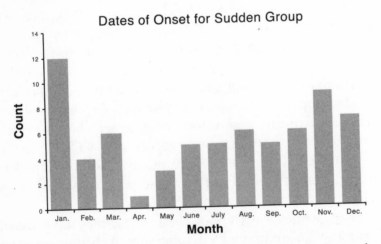

### Dates of Onset for Sudden Group

Patients who have a sudden onset of CFS usually remember the date to the day that their illness began. We asked these patients to tell us the date and found what is called a nonrandom distribution, meaning that the illness started more often in winter months than during the other months of the year.

study, female medical students with systolic pressures less than 100 had a seven-fold increased risk of reporting fatigue five or ten years after completing medical school than med students with higher pressures. This relation did not hold for male students.

Is CFS contagious? People who develop CFS after an infection always worry about this. I have heard stories of close contacts of patients with CFS also developing this illness. Fortunately, however, this does not appear to happen enough to support evidence of contagion. But there have been reports of chronic fatigue occurring in groups of people who had fallen ill with an infectious-type illness at about the same time. One medical article that captured a great deal of interest reported that groups of people living near Lake Tahoe in the mid-1980s developed an illness that I would have labeled "chronic fatigue plus." The Centers for Disease Control, a federally funded group of doctors and researchers who track and try to understand why disease occurs in clusters, were so interested in these mini-epidemics on the California-Nevada border that they established a research team ready to go with the next report of such a problem. But since no other cluster seemed to come soon enough, the project was abandoned.

One mini-epidemic of CFS, although not preceded by infection, did occur in veterans of the 1990–1991 Persian Gulf war. Rates of this illness were approximately three times higher in these veterans than in veterans who never left the United States, and the incidence of illness was also higher in female than in male vets. The mini-epidemic onset of CFS in these veterans suggests that something about serving in the Gulf triggered the illness. The nature of that trigger remains a research question even today.

## Widespread Pain, Bodily Tenderness, and Fibromyalgia

Unlike people whose fatigue begins with flulike symptoms and who often are sent to doctors specializing in infectious diseases, those reporting a slow progression of bodywide pain usually wind up seeing doctors who specialize in rheumatic diseases, problems related to the ligaments or joints. This referral pattern

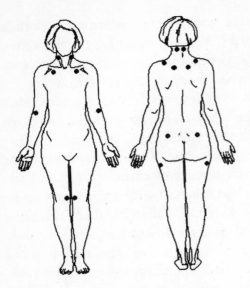

The diagnosis of FM requires a person to have symptoms (widespread pain) and signs (patient reports pain in eleven or more of the eighteen points depicted when pressed with 9 pounds of pressure). One problem with this figure is that it ignores mouth and face pain, which are often part of widespread pain. So in addition to testing these eighteen points for tenderness, I usually test the jaw muscles and other places in the face. Doing this allows me to consider TMD as diagnosis in addition to FM.

started when doctors believed that widespread pain with bodily tenderness (that is, FM) was a disease of the muscles, joints, and ligaments. Research over the past decade has mostly ruled out that possibility, but people with these complaints still fill rheumatologists' offices. Unfortunately, these doctors are often not trained in pain management.

In the same way that doctors try to find a medical cause for severe fatigue, they also try to find a medical cause for widespread pain with tenderness. The reason in both cases is that medical causes may be treatable or even curable. In contrast to the myriad causes of fatigue, substantially fewer disease processes produce widespread pain. So the workup for medical causes of widespread pain and tenderness is easier to do and is substantially shorter than that for severe and long-lasting fatigue. The group that defined FM decided to divide patients into groups with either primary or secondary FM. Primary FM has no medical explanation while secondary FM comes along with another disease, usually rheumatoid arthritis (RA) or systemic lupus erythematosis (SLE).

The diagnosis of FM requires the presence of widespread pain lasting at least three months, plus multiple tender points (see the figure on this page for the location of the tender points). "Widespread" is a qualitative term, but some people really do have pain all over their bodies. It's in less-clear cases that a more specific definition becomes handy. Over time, a consensus developed to define "widespread pain" as pain occurring above and below the waist, on both left and right sides as well as in the chest, neck, or middle to lower back. Although this usually translates into pain in all four quadrants, or quarters, of the body, someone with pain in three areas—for example, the right shoulder, left buttock, and spine— would also satisfy the list for having "widespread pain" and would receive the diagnosis of FM, while someone with pain in the right shoulder, right buttock, and spine would not. In addition to pain, the patient must have tenderness or pain in at least eleven of the eighteen points depicted in the figure on page 60. Obviously, squeezing people hard enough would make just about anyone feel pain, so doctors also decided to set a standard: applying 9 pounds (4 kilograms) of pressure to the area to be tested. In my office, I use a baby scale to teach staff how to push with a pressure of 9 pounds.

Chronic widespread pain occurs twice as often in women as in men (15 percent versus 8 percent). Rates of this complaint tend to increase as women grow older, peaking at 25 percent for women aged sixty to sixty-four. Adding the requirement for multiple tender points magnifies the gender disparity and makes FM a major issue in women's health. For example, FM rates in the city of London, Ontario, were 4.9 percent of all women compared to 1.6 percent of all men. The epidemiologists doing this work extended their study to include Amish people living in rural Ontario. Why? The researchers wanted to see whether a tendency to file lawsuits played a role in FM, since they were concerned that the prospect of large financial rewards might coax patients into claiming severe, widespread pain where lesser pain existed. Lawsuits are rare in the Amish community, making it a good control group for such a study. But the answer proved to be a huge surprise: Rates of FM in Amish women and men were nearly double what they had been in the city. And when FM accompanied a rheumatological disease like SLE, rates more than doubled again. Why would this happen? Surprisingly, no researcher has ever tried to answer this question. But its existence suggests a medical basis for FM.

Besides being a middle-aged woman, other risk factors for developing FM later in life include lower income, less education, and a prior history of lower back pain. Although there is no information as to whether a relation exists among these three factors, one guess would be that women with lower income and less education might do more physically demanding jobs that could lead to injury. Trauma of some sort is commonly reported at the outset of symptoms. The trauma can be from an injury or even following serious surgery.

As people segue from having just widespread pain to having FM, they also start looking more and more like patients with CFS. They develop more problems with fatigue and unrefreshing sleep, and often complain that even minimal exertion produces a dramatic worsening of their fatigue. I will discuss the overlap between these syndromes toward the end of this chapter.

## Mouth and Face Pain and Temporomandibular Disorder

People with FM often complain of pain in the mouth or face, which, if not recognized, can lead to unnecessary dental surgery. Laura Pace was an example. She was a forty-two-year-old professional who had a ten-year history of progressive pain throughout her body. Several years before, she had been given the diagnosis of fibromyalgia, but afterward her doctor told her there was nothing available to help her. A few months before coming to see me, she developed severe pain in the jaw above one of her upper molars. She went to her dentist, who out of desperation did a root canal procedure on the neighboring tooth. The procedure was unsuccessful in relieving the pain, which continued until I began the pain management regimen I will discuss in detail in chapter 7.

Once again, the vagaries of the term *widespread pain* in the textbook definition of fibromyalgia led my patient's physician (and dentist) to guess wrong. The tender points depicted in the figure on page 60 make it seem as if FM is a disease of muscles from the neck down. This is not the case. Forty percent of patients with FM also have pain in their face or mouth when muscles of the face or mouth area are compressed. When face or mouth pain presents by itself, the person goes to the dentist, and dentists have been the primary researchers of temporomandibular disorder (TMD). "Temporo" refers to the temple, while "mandibular" means the jaw. Originally the syndrome was called temporomandibular joint disorder, but researchers learned that quite a few patients with pain in or around their TM joint had pain in the muscles and not in the joint itself. The diagnosis requires the report of spontaneous or chewing-induced pain in the face, mouth, or ears plus tenderness in at least three different muscles with 3 pounds of pressure by the examiner.

My colleague Dr. Karen Raphael has done an epidemiological study of the overlap between FM and TMD. Using a computer to randomly select phone numbers, she identified 2,000 women who provided information over the telephone suggesting that they had either FM, TMD, or both disorders. The rates of FM she found in women were similar to those reported by other researchers: 4.1 percent. And as I indicated previously, 40 percent of these women also had temporomandibular disorder. TMD was found in 13.3 percent of the study group, but only a tenth of them also had FM (so rates of women having both FM and TMD were very low). These results mean that face and jaw pain are common in women with FM but that face pain occurring alone may be a different beast from that occurring with FM. An alternative but very interesting idea is that pain localized to the face and head can lead to the widespread pain indicative of FM. I find that my treatment plan for reducing body pain also helps with face or mouth pain. So my pain management program aims to relieve pain regardless of its location.

## Belly Pain, Altered Bowel Habits, and Irritable Bowel Syndrome

The hallmark of irritable bowel syndrome (IBS) is abdominal pain with a change in bowel habits. My patient Simone Jay provides an example. She was a thirty-six-year-old secretary who came to see me complaining of crampy pain in her lower abdomen, leading to an urge to use the toilet. When she did, she had loose stools, but the cramps were relieved. In addition, she reported having occasional bouts of constipation, also with belly pain. Constipation, Mrs. Jay reported, had become pretty much a normal part of her life, except every so often when an attack of belly pain led to diarrhea instead. And then she happened to contract a rather severe case of food poisoning, which changed the pattern. Now the attacks of pain and diarrhea were occurring much more frequently, as often as once a week. Her case provides two examples. Prior to the food poisoning, she had a quietly simmering case of IBS. Afterward, it became rip-roaring. In contrast to Mrs. Jay's case, some women have no gastrointestinal problems at all but then get an acute GI infection followed by the new onset of IBS.

Because no specific test exists to diagnose IBS, the medical community has used the same tactic as with the other unexplained illnesses, turning to a group of experts to determine a set of clinical criteria needed for diagnosis. Because all the experts specialized in dysfunction of the digestive system, the major symptoms used to identify IBS are those related to the function of the bowel. To set out criteria, one group of researchers determined how often certain symptoms in people with medically caused bowel disease compared to symptoms in people whose bowel symptoms had no obvious medical cause. They found several symptoms to be much less common in the group with medically unexplained disease: relief of pain after bowel movement; looser stools at the onset of pain; more frequent bowel movements at the onset of pain; abdominal distention; stools mixed with mucus; and the feeling that the bowels were not empty at the end of the bowel movement. The group made the decision to diagnose IBS when two of these symptoms were present. A follow-up study checked to see just how well these criteria did in identifying people with IBS. The researchers gave a gastrointestinal symptom questionnaire to 1,344 introductory psychology students and found that 19 percent of the women and 10 percent of the men fulfilled criteria for IBS. While sex was important for the diagnosis, race was not; Caucasians and African Americans had very similar rates of IBS.

Once this initial definition was established, other groups of expert physicians met to decide whether these criteria did a good job in differentiating "cases" of IBS from the normal variation in bowel symptoms that might occur in anyone. They found two problems: the criteria didn't consider any duration of symptoms before the diagnosis could be made, and they also did not require abdominal pain, even though the original group recognized it as probably the most common symptom of IBS. That pain can occur anywhere in the abdomen but most often is found in the pelvic area, either on both sides or only one. Subsequent consensus groups modified the original criteria accordingly. The most recent definition of IBS, called the Rome II criteria, is at least twelve weeks, not necessarily consecutive, in the past twelve months of abdominal discomfort or pain that has two of the following features:

- Relieved with defecation; and/or
- Onset associated with a change in frequency of stool; and/or
- Onset associated with a change in form or appearance of stool

One recent study sought to determine how use of each of these different clinical case criteria affected the ability to diagnose IBS. The researchers sent questionnaires about abdominal symptoms and bowel habits to a large group of people living in Sydney, Australia. A total of 14 percent of respondents met the criteria for IBS using the earlier, more liberal criteria, while only 7 percent met the new criteria for IBS from the Rome II case definition. The most important point made by this study is that IBS is very common. To me, that is much more important than the observation that how one defines IBS influences the rate at which it is found.

One of the problems concerning IBS is that symptoms often wax and wane a great deal, a difference from CFS/ICF and FM, where symptoms tend to be long-term and do not fluctuate as dramatically. One study followed 122 IBS patients over a four-month period, using a telephone method allowing patients to report symptoms on a daily basis. Although most patients reported at least one IBS symptom on half of the reported days, it was unusual for the patient to report being bothered by all possible symptoms on any particular day. Indeed the patients reported feeling fine for a while, then having problems with IBS symptoms, and then feeling fine again. On the average, the patients reported having twelve episodes of symptoms over the four-month study period. In general, people reported their symptoms to be moderately severe during these episodes, with pain and bloating lasting an average of five days and altered bowel habits up to two days. Most patients cycled back and forth between a few days with symptoms and a few days without symptoms.

The effect these symptoms have on quality of life is considerable. A group of IBS patients reported having more pain and fatigue and a greater impairment of normal social functioning than a group of chronically ill patients with kidney disease requiring dialysis. This impact often translates into taking off from work and/or visits to the doctor.

I say "and/or" because not all patients with symptoms consistent with the diagnosis of IBS take their problem to the doctor. One study in Minnesota found that only half the patients with IBS actually went to the doctor because of their symptoms. The things that led a person to become a patient were all related to abdominal pain. If it was severe and affected daily life, if attacks occurred once a week or more, or if the episodes of pain lasted for more than two hours, the symptomatic person would probably see a doctor and become a patient. Research has also shown that people who tend to be pessimistic seek medical care more often than those who take a positive view of events, so we know that, generally speaking, psychological factors are important in determining whether an individual decides to become a patient. But that doesn't change the underlying causes of IBS, which are identical whether or not a patient decides to go to the doctor with a complaint. This dissociation between psychological distress, the decision whether to see a doctor, and the underlying process causing IBS is probably responsible for the fact that IBS patients who do seek medical care may often be anxious or depressed.

## Sensitivity to Odors and Multiple Chemical Sensitivity

Multiple chemical sensitivity (MCS) is the last syndrome I will cover, and the unexplained illness we know the least about. Doctors have known for many years that exposure to toxic chemicals like asbestos or cleaning fluids can make people sick. But some people develop medical symptoms after moving into new buildings, leaving doctors stumped about the cause. Eventually, these patients were said to have developed "sick building syndrome," another medically unexplained illness. The symptoms included eye, nose, or throat irritation; dry cough; dry or itchy skin; dizziness and nausea; difficulty concentrating; fatigue; and sensitivity to odors. Usually the symptoms went away when the individual left the environment, but in some cases the symptoms persisted and would be made substantially worse by exposure to strong odorants, such as detergents, perfumes, newsprint, and insecticides. Patients with these complaints were said to have multiple chemical sensitivity. Though many MCS cases seem to start with an identifiable trigger (like working in a new building), some have no apparent trigger. So far, no good consensus definition for this condition exists.

Based on the available literature, I have tried to arrive at a way of diagnosing this condition. Patients with these complaints often seek care from doctors specializing in a field called environmental or occupational medicine. I'm not that kind of doctor, so I don't see patients whose primary complaint has to do with odors and chemicals. But I do see many patients with problems related to pain or fatigue, of course, so I can determine rates of MCS in people who may be unaware that they have chemical sensitivity.

Here the history is the thing; there are no rule-outs or exclusions. I diagnose MCS if a person mentions being sensitive to more than two chemicals or odors and says that exposure to these chemicals produces symptoms in two different bodily systems—for example, making him or her feel nauseated but also interfering with concentration. The clincher is when the person goes out of his or her way to avoid exposure to the odors. But of course, the strong relation between the symptoms and the avoidance of them is not a surprise. Who wants to get sick?

My experience is clearly different from that of doctors of environmental medicine. Only a few of my patients report an acute exposure that initiated their symptoms. The rest split into two groups: one that dates chemical sensitivity to a time at or after they had developed their other symptoms (such as chronic fatigue), and the other saying their chemical sensitivity dates back many years. The presence of this second group leads me to wonder whether, for some people, chemical sensitivity, even if mild, is a risk factor for developing fatigue or pain later in life. While I don't have an answer to that question, it's clear that there is some overlap among CFS, FM, IBS, and MCS.

## The Question of Syndromic Overlap

When people complain of severe fatigue, they usually have other symptoms as well. How does that affect the diagnoses of different medically unexplained syndromes? One group looked at that exact question when they compared twenty-five patients with CFS and twenty-two patients with FM. There was a moderate amount of overlap among the diagnostic categories: 20 percent of the CFS patients had FM, while 64 percent of the FM patients had CFS; and interestingly over 75 percent of patients in both groups had IBS. But there were some differences. Fevers and sore throats were much less common in FM than in CFS, while the pain in FM was better relieved by heat or massage than was the pain in CFS.

The overlap among syndromes is important for two reasons. First and foremost, it is confusing for patients and physicians alike. A patient whose primary concern is widespread joint pain, as we've already seen, may be referred to a rheumatologist, who may miss other symptoms—such as constant fatigue—or assume them to be less urgent. A doctor whose patient complains of abdominal cramps and altered bowel movements may assume that the patient's other symptoms (pain elsewhere in the body, for example) all stem from the "original" cause: something wrong in the gastrointestinal tract. But overlap among the various "unexplained" illness syndromes turns out to be one of their main characteristics.

Additionally, the significance of syndromic overlap has implications about their cause or etiology. For example, an important idea driving my own research is that a patient with only one medically unexplained illness may have a very different illness, with a different cause, from that of another patient who has two or more of the illnesses we've been discussing. The exact opposite idea is that these syndromes are just variations of one another where "somatic symptoms are incorrectly attributed to serious abnormality, reinforcing the patient's belief that he or she has a serious illness"—in other words, that all these patients are somatizers who really have "nothing wrong" with them. Looked at from my perspective, the ratio of biological to psychological factors may weigh more toward the biological for a patient with CFS alone and more toward the psychological for another patient with all of the syndromes I have discussed to this point. In fact, the more overlapping illnesses, the higher the rate for depression or anxiety disorder: for CFS alone, rates were 44 percent; for CFS with MCS or with FM, about 60 percent, and for CFS with both FM and MCS, 85 percent.

So I think it is very important to evaluate every patient for each of these other syndromes. My group has done careful studies of patients who had CFS only, CFS with FM, and CFS, FM, and MCS. As expected, we found that the typical woman with CFS often had one of the other diagnoses too. While nearly 40 percent of my patients had CFS alone, somewhat fewer also had FM, somewhat fewer yet had MCS instead, and only 16 percent had both FM and MCS in addition to their CFS. As you might expect, we found that patients with both CFS and FM reported more pain than patients with CFS alone, and had more difficulty getting through physical activities. In contrast, those with CFS alone were twice as likely to report a sudden onset of their illness and to have objective evidence for cognitive problems than those with CFS plus FM. The increased rate of a sudden onset correlates with the fact that getting infectious mononucleosis greatly increases the risk for developing CFS or idiopathic chronic fatigue but not for IBS or FM. In contrast, having a severe GI infection increases the risk for developing IBS but not CFS or ICF. If all these illnesses were the same, the type of infection would not matter.

What do these facts suggest? CFS, by itself, may be a different disease from CFS that's accompanied by other medically unexplained illnesses. And data exist from an excellent research group at DePaul University to support this idea. Using a computer to generate phone numbers, the DePaul researchers called people living in Chicago and identified those who complained of chronic fatigue; they then compared these respondents' symptoms to those of a group of healthy people. Next they brought the patients into the laboratory and had them undergo medical examinations to determine if they had CFS, FM, and/or IBS. After the patients answered a large number of questions, the researchers asked themselves three major questions about the patients' responses: (1) Could all the symptoms be explained by one general construct called functional somatic distress? The answer was no. (2) Could all the symptoms be explained by the presence of depression and anxiety? The answer again was no. (3) Did the symptoms appear in ways suggesting that CFS, FM, IBS, depression, and anxiety were inherently different from one another? The answer was yes. This statistical approach indicates that the symptoms of each of these five clinical conditions differ in key ways from one another. This is strong evidence that despite some overlap among these syndromes, they do differ from one another. Thus, although specific diagnostic lab tests do not yet exist to distinguish CFS, FM, and IBS from one another, their different symptoms strongly suggest to me the existence of various mechanisms within the body that cause each syndrome.

To sum up, following are the diagnostic rules for each of the syndromes I have detailed in this chapter:

- Chronic fatigue syndrome (CFS). New onset of medically unexplained fatigue lasting at least six months and producing a substantial decrease in activity plus substantial problems lasting at least six months with at least four of the following symptoms: unrefreshing sleep, sore throat, tender lymph glands, achy muscles, achy joints, headache, brain fog, increased symptoms after minimal exertion.
- Idiopathic chronic fatigue (ICF). Either less substantial fatigue plus the same number of symptoms as in CFS or fatigue producing a substantial decrease in activity plus fewer than four of the symptoms as in CFS.
- Fibromyalgia (FM). Widespread pain (often in all four quadrants of the body) lasting at least three months plus tenderness in eleven or more of the points seen in the figure on page 60.

- Irritable bowel syndrome (IBS). Abdominal discomfort or pain lasting at least three months with at least two of the following features:

  Relieved with defecation

  Onset associated with a change in frequency of stool

  Onset associated with a change in form or appearance of stool

- Multiple chemical sensitivity (MCS). Complaint that at least two different odors produce symptoms in at least two different bodily systems plus efforts to avoid those odors.

I evaluate every new patient in my practice for each of these syndromic diagnoses because they let me test my idea that one of these syndromes alone may have a different cause from several of these syndromes occurring together.

A few words about what's next. In chapter 4, you'll learn how to determine whether your doctor is right for you and how to get a second opinion, if either you or your doctor deems this worth while. Chapter 5 focuses on depression, which makes every illness worse. Depression is also relevant because many doctors mistake its symptoms for those of the symptoms we've been discussing in this chapter. Even if you think depression is not a problem for you, I would urge you to skim through chapter 5. And if you have concerns that depression could be contributing to your illness, please read it in detail because I lay out current treatment strategies. Once we've completed our discussion of communication between you and your doctors, and explored depression, we can get into the heart of this book: treatment techniques that can help you get well.

# 4

# When to Seek a Second Opinion and When to See a Specialist

You are a twenty-eight-year-old mother of a five-year-old son, and you work as a dental hygienist. Your days are incredibly busy: you send your boy off to all-day kindergarten, put in a full day's work, and then come home and do what has to be done to keep your house and family in order. Your plate is full. Then, all of a sudden, you become ill. You feel like you have the flu. You're bleary eyed and totally wiped out with a fever, a bad sore throat, and swollen glands the size of golf balls in your neck. You are, in fact, presenting exactly the symptoms that doctors see in 25 percent of cases that turn out to be difficult to diagnose. You go to see your doctor, who examines you and draws some blood. She calls you a few days later to report that your white blood cell count is a bit low; this low count suggests the presence of a viral infection. When you ask her if you have mononucleosis, she responds, "Your symptoms are exactly the same as those of a person with mono, but your blood tests don't support that diagnosis."

So you know what you *don't* have. Now what? The doctor said to rest, drink a lot of fluids, and take aspirin for the fever—a set of prescriptions that you could have come up with on your own. You might have added one for chicken soup!

Time goes on, and you don't feel any better. A week passes, then three. You remain wiped out, unable to work or care for your home, and you can barely get your child off to school. You make another appointment with your doctor. She examines you and tells you that the lymph glands in your neck are much smaller than they were at your last visit and that this is an important sign of improvement, but you still feel awful. You feel slammed with fatigue, feverishness, achiness all over, sleeplessness, and a fuzzy-headed feeling. Your doctor explains that even though you don't have mono, you probably have something like it, and these viruses often take up to a few months to disappear.

You go home and drag on. The weeks slip away, and one day you realize that you've been sick for a few months. You speak with your doctor again, and she tells you that there really is nothing more she can do for you. You just have to wait it out. While telling you this, she seems a bit defensive and curt. You ask her to recommend someone who might be able to offer a second opinion. Suddenly she seems more positive, and tells you that this is a good idea.

## Asking for a Second Opinion

In this case, you—not your doctor—initiated a referral for a second opinion. Patients are often uncomfortable about asking for another doctor's input. They sense that some doctors think that a referral is a mark against them; it shouldn't be. In fact, as soon as a primary-care doctor feels uncomfortable because a patient's condition seems to evade diagnosis, he or she should refer the patient to another doctor for a second opinion. It is surprising, though, just how often physicians hold off on doing so. In this example, your doctor may feel a bit relieved that you raised the issue, and you will certainly be better off with a second opinion.

If you're on the fence about whether to seek a second opinion, ask yourself these questions:

1. Weeks have passed and you're still sick. When you see your doctor again, does he or she fail to answer your questions?
2. Do you think that your doctor is brushing you off?
3. Does your doctor say that he or she can't help you?
4. Does your doctor tell you there is "nothing wrong" with you?

If the answer to any of these questions is yes, then it's time to seek a second opinion. The mechanics of getting a second opinion depend on either the type of medical insurance you have or your willingness to pay out of pocket. If you belong to an HMO, your primary care provider acts as a "gatekeeper," the only person who can grant you access to medical services beyond those he or she provides (including specialists). So the actual referral has to come from your doctor, even though you asked him or her to provide it. Another limitation of the HMO is that the doctor you would like to see may not be on the HMO's approved doctor list. Some patients bypass these problems by simply deciding to pay for the second opinion themselves. If, on the other hand, you have what is called a "traditional" medical insurance plan, then you can decide when to get that second opinion and whom to consult, paying whatever portion of the charges your insurer doesn't cover.

## Where You Should Go for a Second Opinion

The credentials and expertise of your family doctor will influence your decision about the kind of doctor you see next.

### If Your Doctor Is a Family Doctor

You should find an internist for a second opinion if your doctor is a family practitioner. The difference between these two types of doctors lies in the breadth of their training. Family doctors have very broad training that prepares them to help patients with common conditions such as lacerations, colds, and pregnancy. Internists, in contrast, receive a more focused education in medical problems with no further training in surgery or obstetrics at all. Finding a good internist is simple. Ask your friends, call the department of medicine in your neighborhood hospital, or look in the yellow pages for a doctor who has accreditation—that is, who is "board certified"—in internal medicine.

### If Your Doctor Is an Internist

If you're already seeing an internist, then it does not make sense to go to another internist. Instead, you should ask about a referral to a specialist (or decide to refer yourself if your insurance allows this). In this case, a second opinion is important because your internist may not know what your problem is. He or she might say so, but might instead give you a diagnosis—like fibromyalgia—just for the sake of giving you a diagnosis.

How can you tell if your doctor is doing this? If your doctor makes a diagnosis of fibromyalgia, he or she should be prepared to discuss a treatment plan with you. This plan, like the one I will outline in chapter 7, should include a set of steps to help you manage your discomfort. Your doctor may not provide you with a plan that is as detailed as the one in this book, but he or she should be able to describe an overall approach. A treatment plan that's limited to a single drug for pain (like Celebrex or Motrin) often is inadequate because these medicines alone are less likely to bring about substantial relief than a more comprehensive plan. If your physician does not offer you more than a prescription, ask for a referral to a specialist.

A doctor's lack of familiarity with illnesses like fibromyalgia does not necessarily mean that he or she is dismissing your concerns. Here again, the issue is depth of training. Internists know a great deal about common illnesses like high blood pressure, asthma, and heart disease. However, they often do not have adequate training in methods to reduce chronic, widespread pain. There is just too much to learn.

A similar problem exists with the symptom of fatigue. Quite often, a second doctor whose training is more specialized will be able to get to the root of your problem and will be able to help you manage it. Next, let's look at the types of specialists that your doctor may refer you to, and at the ways in which he or she will decide where to send you for a referral.

## Types of Specialists You May See

Your pattern of symptoms will determine the kind of specialist you should see next.

### For Fatigue, Sore Throat, Tender Glands, and Fever

Let's say that you are the twenty-eight-year-old dental hygienist in the earlier example. Your doctor did not find abnormalities during your exam or in your blood tests, so he or she probably will refer you to a specialist. Your illness began with an infection and your symptoms appear to be those of someone with a chronic infection, so your doctor may choose to send you to an infectious disease expert.

When you see this type of specialist, be sure to tell him or her about all of your symptoms, including malaise, throat pain, swollen glands, and a fever. If you have had a fever (an oral or ear temperature exceeding 100 degrees), chart your temperature over the course of several days or weeks—however long your fever persists. Record your temperatures upon awakening in the morning and before you go to sleep at night. Remember to take your temperature before you brush your teeth or smoke a cigarette, as these activities may change your temperature reading. When it's time to see the specialist, bring this chart with you.

Although the infectious disease specialist will do a complete evaluation, including all the blood tests listed in chapter 2, he or she may rule out the possibility of an infection if your temperature chart is normal and blood tests also show no abnormalities. The specialist has gone through a diagnostic algorithm and has come up shorthanded. But one can diagnose chronic fatigue syndrome (CFS) or its less severe counterpart, idiopathic chronic fatigue (ICF), without any such abnormalities. If the doctor knows the requirements for diagnosing either of these, he or she may go on to make one of those diagnoses.

## For Muscle Aches and Joint Pain

Let's say you are another twenty-eight-year-old whose illness started with a fever, a sore throat, swollen glands, and body aches. Eventually the symptoms of a potential infection—fever, sore throat, and tender glands—go away, and you're left with continuing achiness. Your discomfort gradually gets worse, so that any little motion causes you to feel horrible pain all over your body and extreme tenderness to the touch.

This problem with widespread pain also can start by itself, without any of the symptoms of infection. When it starts this way, months or even years may pass before the ailment is severe enough to slow you down. Whether the pain begins with other symptoms or by itself, when you have gone to your doctor more than once complaining of widespread pain, he or she may refer you to a rheumatologist—a specialist in conditions of the muscles, joints, and fibrous tissue. The rheumatologist will try to rule out the possibility that you have rheumatoid arthritis (RA) or systemic lupus erythematosis (SLE). If he or she cannot make this diagnosis, the doctor may diagnose fibromyalgia (FM).

Although FM is probably the most common diagnosis a practicing rheumatologist makes, the key to helping FM patients is pain management. Most rheumatology training programs do not cover this type of therapy adequately. Moreover, although people with widespread pain often wind up seeing rheumatologists, FM is not a rheumatological disease; that is, it is not a disease of the joints. For this reason, and because it's often beyond the limits of their training, many rheumatologists are uncomfortable treating patients for FM. If a rheumatologist says that you have FM but has little else to offer, ask him or her if you need a referral to a pain management specialist.

## For Abdominal Discomfort or Diarrhea

What if your symptoms are a little different? Say you're another twenty-eight-year-old woman, a teacher. You wake up one day with severe crampy pain in your abdomen, nausea, and bad diarrhea. You also have some of the other symptoms of the first twenty-eight-year-old: a fever, horrible fatigue, achiness all over, messed up sleep, and a foggy brain. Two or three months later, many of your symptoms have finally disappeared, but you still feel wiped out and you still have abdominal pain and diarrhea. At this point, your doctor will probably refer you to a gastroenterologist, an expert in illnesses of the stomach and intestines.

Be sure to tell the gastroenterologist if your upset stomach and crampy pain can be relieved by a bowel movement, or if you have occasional diarrhea and then constipation. These symptoms point to irritable bowel syndrome (IBS), but the specialist will most likely diagnose IBS only if he or she cannot find another cause for your symptoms. To do this, the gastroenterologist may order tests including an X-ray series to view your bowel. If the results of these tests do not reveal another gastrointestinal problem, you may have IBS. The good news is that new drug treatments are available for this disorder—specifically for women whose symptoms are either predominantly diarrhea or predominantly constipation.

### For Face or Jaw Pain

IBS is an example of isolated, or regional, pain that occurs in the belly. Another type of isolated pain may be limited to the face and jaw. If you experience this form of pain and chewing is uncomfortable, you will probably visit your dentist before you visit your doctor.

If you go to a dentist because of mouth, tooth, or jaw pain, he or she may well recognize that you do not have a dental problem but rather a regional pain problem; that is, you may have temporomandibular disorder (TMD). However, some dentists think that they can cure the problem by pulling teeth or performing a root canal. I have seen many patients who have had these procedures yet noticed very little improvement. So, if your dentist suggests one of these procedures because of TMD (as opposed to an appropriate dental problem, like a cavity or root decay) and refers you to an oral surgeon, beware.

Often when I see and question such patients, they also complain of pain elsewhere in the body. Because their oral pain is so severe, however, they focus on that aspect of their problem and wind up having dental surgery. As I explained in the last chapter, however, TMD may not be isolated at all but actually can be part of a broader problem with pain. If your dentist sends you to a TMD expert who recommends a bite plate or some other prosthesis, it's certainly worth a try. It could at least relieve some of the mouth or jaw pain, and is less permanent than losing a tooth. If he or she wants to drill or pull teeth, however, you should get a second opinion first. I would suggest going to someone other than a dentist, perhaps a physician who specializes in FM or pain management.

### For Unrelenting Chronic Pain

Speaking of pain management, if you suffer from unrelenting pain in your gut, head, or throughout your body, and this pain continues despite your doctor's best efforts, he or she may refer you to an expert in pain management. Managing pain often requires various approaches, so most specialists in pain management work in centers, with an entire team of experts. One doctor may have expertise in relieving pain with injections into muscle or into ligaments near the backbone. He or she also may be a specialist in surgical approaches to pain. Another may be an expert in hypnosis or in acupuncture, and another may be an expert in the use of medicines to relieve pain. Pain management centers also frequently employ counseling professionals who help people cope with the emotional consequences of having to live with chronic pain.

## Questions to Ask Your Primary Care Doctor or Internist

Each of these referral tracks makes sense, but whether you will get any satisfaction when it is your doctor who makes the referral will depend just as much on the specialist's nature as on his or her specialty. If the doctor is curious, scientifically oriented, and empathetic, you will have a more satisfying consultation than if he or she is interested only in getting to the next patient. Sad to say, some doctors don't care much about the latest scientific advances, unless they pertain directly to their own very narrow specialty. Others are too busy to keep up with these advances, and others are just cold fish when it comes to caring about patients.

Often, the key to finding the most appropriate and helpful specialist is being able to trust your primary-care provider to steer you toward the right one. I can't emphasize enough how important it is for you to have a primary-care provider with whom you feel comfortable. Being able to have a meaningful two-way conversation with anyone—including your doctor—requires this sense of comfort. Few people feel completely at ease with a new acquaintance; it takes time to build any relationship. Doing so is impossible if you use a "doc-in-a-box"—an urgent-care center whose medical staff changes from one day to the next—and not very easy, either, if you belong to an HMO where you seem to end up with a different primary-care physician each time you show up for an appointment. It is possible, however, to build a comfortable relationship if you have a primary-care doctor who cares for all your medical problems, especially if you have seen this doctor for colds or annual Pap smears over the years.

Patients often tell me they see their illness as so complex that they've decided to avoid their primary-care doctor altogether, managing their illness as best they can on their own. This is an unfortunate decision. Some people do make remarkably good case managers, but almost all who take this course of action are really shortchanging themselves. Although you may think that the primary-care doctor's job is just taking care of sore throats and colds, the role changes in the face of chronic illness. Then the *primary* job of the primary-care provider is to coordinate your care: to be sure you see the right specialist; to be sure you are getting the right medicines at the right doses; and to be sure you do not fall between the cracks produced by seeing a specialist expert in diseases in one part of your body and then another specialist expert in diseases of another part of your body, neither of whom may have the time to talk to each other.

Having someone in charge of all your medical problems allows you to be the patient and not your own doctor. I can't emphasize this enough: having a primary-care doctor is crucial. Once you do, you can decide whether your physician is the right one for you or if you need to try again. You can find such a provider no matter what your address, because primary-care providers constitute the largest group of doctors in the United States. Having a long-term relationship with that person will allow you to feel comfortable asking him or her questions like the following:

- Why are you referring me to this specialist rather than to a different type of specialist?
- Do you know anything about the specialist's training and experience?
- Is the doctor affiliated with a medical school? (If so, this is often a sign that the doctor has innate curiosity and an interest in learning.)
- Do you think the specialist will have the time to think about me and my problem or will he or she be in a rush?

By asking such questions, you may trigger your doctor's thinking so that he or she gives more consideration to the referral. Your doctor may even wind up giving you a different name.

## Qualities to Look For in a Specialist

Okay, your physician has referred you to a specialist, you've discussed what your doctor hopes that specialist can do for you, and perhaps you've even learned more about the specialist's practice or research interests by doing a search online. Now it's time to go to your appointment. Here are some questions that might help you to learn even more about this expert. You might ask:

- Do you see many patients like me?
- What can you do to help me? (If the doctor says, "Nothing, because there is nothing wrong with you," you need to find another doctor.)
- Is there anyone besides you whom I should see?
- Have you seen good results in cases like mine? (Again, a reply of no would suggest the need to find another doctor.)
- Is your office willing to help me with insurance forms? Can your office help me deal with the paperwork necessary to allow me get some time off from work to rest, if needed?

After the first visit, you must ask yourself:

- Do I feel better after seeing this specialist?
- Did this doctor ignore my concerns or make me feel rejected? (If so, you need to find another physician.)

Remember, even the best specialist won't reach a diagnosis or produce major symptom reduction on the first visit. But it's worthwhile to ask yourself whether your new specialist paid attention to you and gave you hope.

As I said in chapter 1, you're a consumer paying for a service—in this case, your specialist's advice. If he or she does not answer your questions or meet your needs, most health insurance carriers will allow you to look for another doctor who will. Physicians sometimes forget that you are paying them to help you. You have a right to get your money's worth; if you find that you are not, you should take your business elsewhere.

## Find a Doctor Who Gives You Enough Time

Other factors may influence your feelings about being on the same page with a specialist, and these factors may also affect the outcome of your relationship with him or her. The first thing that may work against the success of your consultation with any specialist is managed care. Managed care has changed medicine from being patient-centric to being time-centric. Medicine in the twenty-first century is run more and more like industry. Managers of managed-care medical practices treat patients as if they are widgets on an assembly line. In fact, for some, the word *patients* has disappeared and *customer* has replaced it. That form of treatment may have made you uncomfortable in the care of your primary doctor, who may have had you out the door at the end of fifteen minutes, even though you really had not communicated your concerns or learned how to deal with them.

In modern medicine, few initial consultations are booked for longer than one hour. Medical accountants have rightly calculated that nearly every patient can receive a total and comprehensive evaluation in this amount of time. The operative phrase, though, is "nearly every patient." As soon as a doctor has no landmarks to follow as to diagnosis and treatment, the critical thing needed is time: time to really understand what is going on with the patient; time for doctor and patient to converse so that both can wind up on the same page; and time for the doctor to think through the best approach to the patient's problems. The bottom line is, once again, that you're paying for your doctor's time. If you don't feel that your doctor is listening to you—or even taking enough time to hear what you're saying—then you need to find another doctor.

## Seek Out a Female Doctor

Two decades ago, most doctors were men. Things are different today. Nearly half of the physicians who graduate from medical school are women. This may come as something of a surprise, since I'm a male doctor, but I suggest that you look for a female physician. Studies show that many patients find female physicians to be better listeners and explainers, less likely to dismiss your symptoms than a male doctor would. The differences may be even more acute if you're a woman. My colleagues and I have found that women with CFS feel less stigmatized by female doctors than by their male counterparts. Of course, there are exceptions to these findings, so you need not despair if you can't find a physician who is female. Male physicians who listen and care can do the job just as well, and hundreds of my patients can attest to that.

## Look for the Three Cs

When you seek a second opinion, keep your antennae up. Look for a doctor who makes you feel comfortable, even though you may be apprehensive about seeing a new physician. This apprehension is very common. In fact, a patient's nervousness in a doctor's office commonly leads to what physicians call white coat hypertension, a condition where your blood pressure shoots up the moment you approach a doctor's office, even though it may be normal at home and even at work. But I'm talking about whether the doctor actually makes you feel more comfortable, especially after you've sat and talked for a while. It's the doctor with what I like to call the three Cs who can do that—a doctor who is *compassionate*, *caring*, and *creative* in helping you feel better. You can view the doctor with the three Cs as the opposite of the one I discussed in chapter 1 with the three Bs.

Feeling pressed for time is no antidote to discomfort. When I see a new patient, I schedule more than an hour for the initial visit, so I have enough time to gather all the information I need without having to hurry. I do everything I can think of to make a patient comfortable. That's why I'm so surprised when a patient tells me of nervousness at being in my office for the first time. I try constantly to find ways to do a better job in this regard, and I'm not doing this just to be polite. When a patient leaves the office of a doctor who does not take such care to put him or her at ease, that patient usually feels worse than she did coming in. That outcome surely is not what a doctor hopes for. Conversely, when leaving the office of a doctor with the three Cs, the patient usually feels better.

Following the three Cs is key. Just helping a patient feel comfortable enough to tell me he or she is anxious being in my office is a step toward reducing anxiety and making the person feel better about the consultation. And for the patient, finding physicians and specialists who exhibit these three qualities is one of the first steps on the road to recovery.

### Seek Out a Curious Doctor

I can even add a fourth C to the list. In addition to being patient and empathetic, a good doctor is *curious*. The curious physician cares about understanding a person's illness. He or she loves being a doctor: sitting and talking with patients about their problems; trying to understand the nature of those problems; and trying to come up with some sort of intervention to help. Essentially the job of a physician is to be a medical detective. A really curious physician will listen to a patient's concerns and then develop a logic trail that leads to a beneficial answer. The goal is to figure out why the patient is sick and either to cure the illness or to reduce the symptoms so that the person can manage to live with them.

Unfortunately, lack of time is once again the enemy. Some doctors who are employees of managed-care companies simply do what they have to do to finish the day at five o'clock. For such physicians, the practice of medicine is not much different from the job of a toll collector on a busy highway. Their medical curiosity has burned out, and they won't have enough interest to figure out a complex medical problem.

Your antennae should alert you to a doctor who is bored with medicine. One clue is if he or she is engaged in medical research; a critical quality for success in research is curiosity. A doctor who also conducts research will view *you* through a research lens. You may seem interesting just because your case is a little more difficult to solve. What you say to such a physician may spark ideas that he or she can put to the test in the laboratory; or perhaps the doctor/researcher is already conducting research to which your case lends itself. Patient contact drives the research of such physicians; they have a vested interest in hearing you out beyond their usual desire to help patients.

Doctors who see patients as well as doing research may have published articles on cases or symptoms just like yours, and publishing articles is one way they advance in stature. You can find out easily on the Internet whether a certain doctor has contributed to the medical literature; go to www.ncbi.nlm.nih.gov/PubMed. This is the Web address of the National Library of Medicine, and many taxpayer dollars have been spent making scientific and medical literature more accessible through this site. Enter a doctor's name, like smith-jones j (while you are at it, you can try natelson bh). The search engine will immediately present you with a list of the person's scientific papers.

Practicing doctors rarely have time for research; their practice is their thing. And very often, a practitioner does not have the facilities needed for research: access to an electronic medical library, other scientists, sensitive equipment, or statisticians who can help interpret scientific results. Nine times out of ten, these facilities are found in medical schools. One way to find a doctor with scientific curiosity is to check the faculty of a medical school near you. Another advantage of finding a doctor who works in a medical school is that, unlike other practitioners in the community, relatively few of these doctors are involved in the kind of managed-care practice that requires them to see a patient every fifteen to twenty minutes. Academic medical practice is often an add-on to the faculty member's other duties. He or she does not have to make a living in practice; such doctors receive a salary both to teach and to see patients. Thus, some academic practitioners can see as many or as few patients as they wish.

Once again, there are exceptions to all generalities. Not all physicians on medical school faculties are endlessly curious. Some have to generate their salary by seeing patients. Some are as burned out by their work or as bogged down by politics and paperwork as some doctors in the nonacademic community. Just as you don't need to despair if you can't find a female doctor, you don't need to despair if you live far from a university medical center. Wonderful, curious doctors are out there, and chances are there is one nearby who can help you. Your task is to go into that first visit with open eyes. Remember to take along the list of questions under

"Qualities to Look for in a Specialist," page 81. Then, if you find that the doctor lacks the curious spark that can lead to a solution to your problem, keep looking for a doctor who has it.

## Look for a Specialist Who Takes an Integrative Approach

In addition to being scientifically oriented, the best specialists take an integrative approach to treating their patients. They focus on the entire person in addition to, but not exclusive of, any particular organ system or disease. That might sound like what a primary-care provider does, but the specialist has much more extensive training in the area of his or her interest. This means they have received training similar to that of the internist or primary-care provider but then continued their studies to learn more about a specific area of medicine, such as rheumatology or infectious diseases. Being integrative means that a doctor should see the patient in a broader scope—as a person with a medical problem living in a community that produces both stress and pleasure, as a person living in an environment that could be pleasant or horrible, and as a person living in a world filled with challenges ranging from terrorism to global warming. Most of us don't think about these global problems every minute of every day, yet we hear about them every time we turn on the evening news or pick up a newspaper. Physicians who take an integrative approach are aware of the many factors influencing our health, including those that lie outside our bodies.

I'm not inventing anything new here. George Engel, a farsighted physician at the University of Rochester, called this the biopsychosocial approach to illness. Engel trained in medicine and then in psychoanalysis in the 1930s, when the concepts of psychosomatic disease were new. In chapter 6, you will see how these concepts changed the way in which doctors viewed the relationship between stress and the body—that is, stress turns on nerves to bodily organs, with pathological consequences. Engel's biopsychosocial model was a direct outgrowth of that line of thought. He believed that psychological and social factors outside of the body play almost as important a role in influencing how a patient feels from day to day as the patient's underlying disease.

Psychosocial factors count whenever chronic illness exists. Your relationship to those closest to you—family and friends—will affect your struggle, whether it is with multiple sclerosis, rheumatoid arthritis, or heart failure. If someone with multiple sclerosis has a husband who is never home and is not supportive, she will have additional trouble coping with her disease as well as a chance of doing worse. If, on the other hand, her spouse is always there for her, she may have trouble walking, but her quality of life will be better for his presence, caring, and concern.

Although a doctor cannot improve a patient's relationships, he or she can be sensitive to them and can try to help patients reduce the consequences of negative aspects of their lives. Sometimes this is as easy as telling a person to take an escape from her life as a sick person to run away with her spouse for a long weekend in the sun. However, if the doctor thinks that "relational therapy" (for example, marriage counseling) is required, this task may be harder, especially if the spouse does not see the need for consulting such a professional.

Despite the fame of Engel's biopsychosocial model, and the work of many of his successors (myself included) to foster his approach, Engel's ideas still haven't reached the mainstream of medical education. Finding a physician who can take an integrative approach to treating a specific symptom you exhibit—like fatigue or chronic pain—may still be a little difficult, unless you happen to live in one of those areas of the country where this approach is more widespread. To see if a doctor where you live follows this approach, type the word "integrative" or "biopsychosocial" into an Internet or National Library of Medicine search engine. You might also try the Web site of a medical university near you. If you get a hit, give that doctor a try.

## Your Visit with a Specialist

Your request for a referral to a specialist was fulfilled, and now you are at the specialist's office.

## What to Watch For

You are in the specialist's office because your doctor thought that an expert in a particular aspect of medicine would have the best chance of helping you. What can you expect to gain by this visit? First, you want to know what is wrong with you; you want a diagnosis. If you turn out to have a medical disease in the specialist's area of competence, your journey is over. Stick with that doctor unless further referrals are necessary for treatments that he or she cannot provide.

*Is the expert too specialized?*   As mentioned earlier in this chapter, the specialist may tell you that your illness does not have a known medical cause and that you have a clinical syndrome. An infectious disease expert may diagnose chronic fatigue syndrome or its less severe counterpart, idiopathic chronic fatigue. A rheumatologist may diagnose fibromyalgia, and a gastroenterologist may diagnose irritable bowel syndrome. Even if the specialist diagnoses one of these syndromes, he or she may not be trained to help you deal with the symptoms that they cause. This is where turning to a specialist for your care has its own potential pitfall: the specialist is an expert in one area of medicine and may be uncomfortable with problems outside of his or her area of expertise. As fond as I am of physicians who work in medical schools (I am one myself), this problem can actually be magnified in academe, where the specialist may not be merely a gastroenterologist but a subspecialist—for example, in diseases of the stomach *only*. Such a "superspecialist" may be less familiar with problems outside of the stomach, in the intestine, than a regular gastroenterologist.

How can you tell if a specialist is too specialized for your needs? He or she may act just like your primary-care doctor, who was not specialized enough. With the now-familiar glazed-over look, the specialist may tell you that he or she doesn't know much about your problem, that he or she can't help you, or that there is "nothing wrong" with you.

*Is the expert willing to address all of your concerns?*   Even if the specialist is not a superspecialist, a problem may remain. An interested and informed rheumatologist may focus on your pain, but he or she may ignore your other complaints. This is a frequent issue for specialists, and some of your concerns can fall through the cracks here. Health problems usually do not occur in a vacuum; they are not always limited to one set of concerns such as widespread pain. For example, one study tracked the medical expenses of patients who had received the diagnosis of FM at least once in a three-year period. Patients in this group—mostly women—had nearly three times more visits to their doctors each year than other claimants. Additional claims for FM were the exception rather than the rule. Instead, these patients sought care for many other concerns, such as backache or abdominal pain, severe fatigue, or problems with sleep, anxiety, and depression.

However, good specialists take an integrative approach to their patients. If you feel that the specialist is considering you simply as the bearer of a specific health problem and not as a whole person, you may need to keep looking for another doctor.

*If you have pain, does the specialist adequately address this problem?*   Chapters 7 and 8 present a lot of detail on treating pain and fatigue; you may want to jump ahead to take a look at that plan. But the bottom line is that most doctors—primary-care doctors as well as specialists—really do not know how to take care of a patient whose major problem is pain. This is true even for many rheumatologists who deal with diseases that frequently cause horrible pain. Many doctors go from prescribing over-the-counter pain medicines like ibuprofen to prescribing narcotics like Percocet when pain continues. This is *not* good medicine. Percocet has no role in the treatment of chronic pain. If you are on your third visit to a doctor and either your pain remains or you are taking Percocet or another such narcotic, you need a referral to a pain management center. They will certainly know how to help you.

*Is your specialist communicating with your primary-care doctor?* If your doctor referred you to the specialist, then it is automatic for the specialist to send the results of the consultation back to him or her. But if you organized your own referral, the specialist has no one with whom to communicate except you. Being knowledgeable about your illness is not the same as having the broad reservoir of medical knowledge of a licensed physician. Therefore, I again urge you to build a relationship with a primary-care provider and make sure that he or she is aware of any appointments you arrange with other doctors. By doing that, you won't have several doctors taking care of several parts of you; instead, you will have one doctor in charge of all of you.

Very strict laws as to the confidentiality of medical records have been in effect since April 2003. Thus, you will have to sign a document authorizing the specialist to release your otherwise confidential information to another party, including your primary-care physician. While you are at it, you might as well ask him or her to send a copy of the letter to you. In contrast to the 1950s and 1960s, when doctors' notes were not available to patients, today you control access to your medical record. You decide who can and cannot see it. In the same vein, you are entitled to have copies of any report or test that pertains to you. After all, you paid for it.

## Trust Your Instincts

Some time after I became a full professor at the New Jersey Medical School, I was involved in a case that dramatically changed the way I thought about medicine and the way we were training young doctors at our medical school. This case alerted me to the dangerous consequences of allowing patients to fall through the cracks of classical medicine. In this instance, the instincts of the patient and her husband prevented a tragic outcome.

The patient was the thirty-six-year-old wife of a practicing neurologist. She had been totally well until she began to notice episodes of rapid heartbeats, or palpitation. She went to her primary-care provider. He evaluated her and found that everything appeared to be normal, including her electrocardiogram. When the problem persisted, her doctor referred her to a local cardiologist.

The cardiologist did a stress test. This test, which demands exhausting exercise, often uncovers cardiac abnormalities. When the results of this test were normal, the cardiologist performed echocardiography, a test that looks inside the heart to evaluate its function. These test results also were normal. Next, the cardiologist tested the patient with a Holter monitor, a beeper-sized machine that records the heart's electrical activity or electrocardiogram for an entire day. While the patient was connected to the monitor, she pushed a button every time she experienced heart palpitations. The only abnormal results of this last test were short bursts of rapid heart rate, or tachycardia. Such bursts commonly occur when a person is exercising or feeling anxious. Because of these test results, the heart doctor's diagnosis was "nothing wrong."

The episodes of jolting, unpleasant heart palpitations continued, and they really disturbed the woman. Her husband called the cardiologist and explained her level of distress to him. The cardiologist advanced her up the referral ladder and sent her to a more specialized specialist—an arrhythmologist, a subspecialist who only sees patients who have bouts of arrhythmia, or abnormal cardiac rhythm. This doctor agreed that the patient's bouts of rapid heartbeats were arrhythmias, but he suggested that they were unrelated to any abnormality in the heart. All people experience similar bouts of rapid heart rate (sinus tachycardia) when they are nervous, scared, or exercising, so this type of arrhythmia is thought to be "normal."

The arrhythmologist told the woman that he agreed with the cardiologist—there was nothing wrong with her. In his letter to the referring cardiologist, he noted that the woman was thin and that her thin chest wall may have made her more aware of her heart beating than would be the case in a heavier-set woman. He didn't say so, but his unwritten diagnosis was that the problem was "all in her head." For an arrhythmia to count for this classically trained subspecialist in cardiology, it had to stem from heart disease. That position made this woman fall through the cracks of classical medicine.

So she was left to her own devices. Fortunately, her husband happened to be a neurologist. She had more and more frequent bouts of tachycardia, and then the woman reported something a bit unusual to her husband. She seemed to have these attacks more reliably just as she was falling asleep or waking up.

When neurologists hear of weird things happening when a person is falling asleep or awakening, they think of seizures. The neurologist called the cardiologist to discuss this idea with him. The cardiologist dismissed his concerns. So the woman's husband took over the management of his wife's illness. He prescribed an anticonvulsant (a medicine that interferes with seizures), and her bouts of sinus tachycardia stopped cold. He then sent her for brain imaging and was aghast to learn that she had a large brain tumor. This brain tumor produced seizures—not the spasmodic twitching usually recognized as a convulsion, but episodes of sinus tachycardia.

There were two terrible things about this case. First, despite the advantage of being a physician's wife, this woman fell through the cracks of classical medicine, was told she had "nothing wrong" with her, and was abandoned as a "crock." With the exception of her husband, the medical profession turned its back on her. Second, her husband was forced into the uncomfortable role of doctoring for his own wife, and ultimately he had to experience the horror of telling her that she had a potentially lethal brain tumor. What would have happened to this woman if her husband hadn't been a physician—and not just any physician but one who had been trained to recognize diseases of the brain?

This woman's trials and tribulations led me to a period of deep introspection. I assumed that this example of one patient falling through the cracks of classical medicine was just the tip of the iceberg. When I started caring for patients with medically unexplained illnesses, I realized that I was right. My patients said that they had seen many doctors who either told them there was "nothing wrong" with them or that their illnesses were all in their heads. If they had not persisted and trusted their instincts (as the woman with the brain tumor and her husband did), they never would have found the help that they were looking for.

You may need to keep looking until you find a doctor who gives you the Harry Truman line "The buck stops here." That doctor will think about you as a person and as a patient with all of your complaints, not just your muscles, your gastrointestinal tract, or your brain. Once you find a doctor who is willing to think outside the standard medical box, the quest for help will end. Many of my patients have seen a dozen doctors before me because the buck did not stop at those doctors' desks.

To review, when you are seeking a second opinion or you need to see a specialist, look first for a female doctor, preferably one who is affiliated with a university medical center. Go to an infectious disease specialist if your illness is characterized mostly by a fever, a sore throat, and swollen glands; to a rheumatologist if your illness is characterized mostly by achy muscles and joints; or to a gastroenterologist if your illness is characterized mostly by stomach pain with constipation or diarrhea. If you suffer from chronic pain, go to a pain management center. But before anything else, make sure that you have a primary-care physician with whom you feel comfortable and who will take an active interest in your health, including working with any specialists you may see. Your primary-care physician may well see critical facts in your overall medical record that one or more specialists have missed. Check out doctors online to see if they've published papers, spoken or written about cases like yours, or been identified as taking an "integrative" approach to care. The National Library of Medicine Web site is among those that will be helpful. Then, when you have your appointment, keep your antennae up to see if you feel cared for and on the same page with the doctor.

Taking care of people who are troubled by medically unexplained pain or fatigue is not rocket science, but it is definitely outside the box of standard medical knowledge and care. Nonetheless, doctors who know a lot about symptom management and illnesses like CFS, FM, and the other medically unexplained syndromes do exist. Your job is to find one. You simply cannot throw up your hands and give up when one doctor after another tells you there is nothing wrong with you. Instead, be your own advocate until you find a thoughtful primary-care provider who will be an advocate for you.

And if your physician says "I don't know," that's not a bad thing, if he or she is willing to learn. Helping the practicing doctor learn about your illness is one reason I wrote this book. As with my last book, *Facing and Fighting Fatigue*, I provide enough detail for your doctor to get up to date quickly so that he or she will be able to take care of you. Just ask him or her to *read the book*. If you and your doctors can't communicate well, you may be tempted to turn your back on traditional medicine and venture into the areas of alternative and complementary medicine, where instead of a physician with a medical degree, you may deal with chiropractic, naturopathic, or homeopathic physicians. Some of these kinds of treatment may indeed play a role in getting you well, but others maybe worthless, expensive, or even dangerous. Charting those troubled waters is the grist for chapter 10.

For now, though, we're going to stay focused on more traditional medicine. Now that you know what you should be looking for in a doctor, how your doctor's mind is likely to operate, and some of the background on unexplained illnesses, we can begin to shift gears. In the next part of the book, we'll talk about illnesses and processes that can either mimic your symptoms or make them a lot worse. Then I'll lay out my own path to wellness. No matter which path to healing you choose, keep your chin up and keep looking for a solution to your illness. Even if a cause and a cure are out of reach for the moment, there are several strategies that you can try to make you feel better. Read on!

# PART TWO

# TOWARD WELLNESS

A Practical Approach to Conquering the "Nothing Wrong" Syndrome

# 5

# Step One: Getting beyond Depression

Let me be clear from the outset. The purpose of this chapter is not to ignore your complaints by calling them depression-related. Instead, please note that depression can be an element explaining why you feel the way you do. You may never have experienced it, but it's possible you may—later on, if you feel beaten down by being ill and not being helped by doctors who simply tell you there's nothing wrong.

It is well worth knowing the facts about depression because depression can bring with it many of the feelings of fatigue and achiness we have discussed to this point. Because of this fact and because women are more likely to experience depression than men, doctors sometimes conclude that people with chronic fatigue or pain don't have a medical problem but instead have either garden-variety depression or some form of masked major depression. In this chapter, we'll look at depression by itself and in combination with fatigue and pain, talk about what happens (or *should* happen) when a patient with medically unexplained illness is also clearly depressed and, finally, we'll discuss how to handle depression if you should experience it.

# Depression: Background and Symptoms

When a patient first visits me with a complaint of severe fatigue or widespread pain, I tell her I hope she is depressed. As you might imagine, this statement usually produces a look of shock. But, strange as it may seem, once depression is identified, it happens to be one illness that today's doctors are good at treating, or even curing. The problem is that depression is hard to recognize, both for the patient and the doctor. It's what I would call a tiptoe disease: it creeps up on people so gradually that they don't see depression for what it really is until it's already become quite advanced. So a patient who can say she's truly depressed has, in a sense, gotten herself a good part of the way toward recovery. That's why it is important for you to recognize the symptoms.

Doctors don't have an easy time recognizing depression either, even if a patient is aware of it and points it out. And some doctors may not treat depression, even though they do recognize it in a patient. Some time ago, doctors participating in a study were told which patients they were seeing for other illnesses also had depression. Amazingly, the doctors just ignored this information even when it was offered to them by other professionals. This, of course, is a major problem, because serious depression can be a lethal disease. In fact, the number two cause of death for women in their twenties and thirties after physical injury is suicide due to depression.

Let me begin with the ABCs of depression itself. As is the case with chronic fatigue syndrome (CFS), fibromyalgia (FM), and irritable bowel syndrome (IBS), psychiatrists have come up with a clinical case definition by consensus. The *Diagnostic and Statistical Manual of Mental Disorders* defines a major depressive episode as requiring "at least 2 weeks during which there is either depressed mood or the loss of interest or pleasure in nearly all activities." These symptoms have to be a change from previous functioning and can't be associated with a recent major loss or cause for bereavement. (For example, if someone in your family dies, you can be expected to feel profound feelings of sadness or even depression, but, given your loss and understandable grief, a doctor wouldn't automatically diagnose depression unless it lasted for a prolonged period of time.)

However, the diagnosis of major depressive disorder—commonly called depression—requires additional symptoms besides these major ones: three more if the patient feels depressed and is experiencing a loss of pleasure or interest, and four more if meeting only one of these two major criteria. These other symptoms include weight loss unrelated to dieting; problems concentrating, thinking, or making decisions; frequent problems with disturbed sleep or too much sleep; markedly increased or decreased activity; fatigue; daily feelings of worthlessness or guilt; and recurring thoughts of death or suicide.

Now that you've seen the list of symptoms that helps define major depressive disorder, perhaps you can understand why doctors may confuse CFS or idiopathic chronic fatigue (ICF) with depression. If someone is sad or down for most of every day of a two-week period, plus has fatigue that forces the curtailment of some activities, plus reports having cognitive problems and disturbed sleep, that person is only one symptom away from the diagnosis of major depressive disorder. At the same time, however, he or she would probably fulfill the case definition for ICF. So which is right? It's important to remember that psychiatrists use more than a depressed mood to diagnose depression. It's these additional symptoms that can lead to diagnostic confusion.

On the other hand, you do not need to be depressed for a doctor to diagnose a major depressive episode. If, instead, you become less interested in things that used to interest you, develop fatigue, become less active, lose some weight, and have difficulty concentrating, a psychiatrist would make the diagnosis of depression. But if you visit an internist instead of a psychiatrist, depression will be the last diagnosis your doctor will be thinking of. And the doctor will nearly always be right and the psychiatrist wrong, because if you had a serious medical condition, you could easily have all of these symptoms as part of it.

When people get sick their behavior can change. For example, when you have the flu, it's not the influenza virus that alters your behavior; it is your body's immune response to the infection that changes the way you feel. To combat the infection, your body releases a tiny amount of highly active immune material called *cytokines*. These function to activate your body's antiviral defense system, but they also make you feel sick. Specifically, they make you exhausted, causing you to sleep longer than usual but in a restless, nonrefreshing way. You lose your appetite, find that you're having problems thinking or concentrating, and may develop achiness all over your body. And because you don't feel well, you're much less interested in things that would usually engage your attention. A psychiatrist finding you in this condition, without running further tests (like taking your temperature or ordering a complete blood count), might conclude that you're depressed. But an internist would probably recognize right away that you had the flu, or some other physical illness. I won't argue with either diagnosis except to point out that medical illness can mimic depression.

The large overlap between the symptoms used to diagnose CFS and those used to diagnose depression may make you wonder why someone with fatigue or widespread pain severe enough to produce a substantial decrease in activity isn't *automatically* depressed. After all, it's normal to feel sad and dejected when a major negative event, such as the loss of a loved one, changes your life. And chronic illness is a major negative event also. When depression occurs after an illness begins, the depression is called reactive. Since depression in this case occurs as a "reaction" to another illness, depression might track illness severity—you might become increasingly depressed if the underlying illness continue to progress.

In fact, our own work on women with CFS makes it clear that illness severity is a major risk factor for depression and/or anxiety. I was disturbed by the fact that the case definition for CFS asked only about the *existence* of symptoms. As far as the Centers for Disease Control (CDC) was concerned, even mild symptoms counted. Because this did not make sense to me in terms of the patients I see, I decided to develop a modification of the case definition designed to identify patients on the severe end of the illness spectrum. About 50 percent of the women we've studied in our federally funded CFS Center have what we call severe CFS. Here's how I define it: fatigue severe enough to reduce activity by more than half from previous normal levels, plus at least one month's worth of substantial, severe, or very severe problems with at least seven symptoms from the 1988 list of minor criteria (I listed those symptoms in chapter 3). While rates of depression or anxiety for women with "less than severe" CFS were in the same range as women with diseases such as multiple sclerosis (MS) or rheumatoid arthritis (RA) (29 percent), rates were over 50 percent in the "severe" group.

One thing that seems to move a woman from the "less than severe" category to the "severe" category of CFS is the addition of fibromyalgia (FM). Women with both CFS and FM are twice as likely to have a problem with depression as those with CFS alone. And when multiple chemical sensitivity (MCS) also exists, rates climb even higher. In fact, we found that only 15 percent of women with CFS, FM, and MCS were free from problems with depression or anxiety. But looking at the other side of this coin, some women with CFS simply don't get the added burden of serious psychiatric problems. The reason not everyone with chronic illness gets depressed relates to specifics about the patient's personality. Women who are optimistic and have no family history of depression tend not to experience long periods filled with sadness, tears, and negative thoughts. Yes, chronic illness is demoralizing, and many of my patients—even though not clinically depressed—have bad days when they feel down in the dumps. But for these particular women, something pleasant or positive eventually happens, and their mood lightens. There is a difference between being temporarily demoralized by illness and being really depressed. Figuring out whether depression is present and then treating it are two of my major goals. When I diagnose depression in a person with medically unexplained illness, I am more committed than ever to wiping out the depression with the goal of reducing the severity of the medical symptoms.

## Is All Depression the Same?

We have compared a group of women who had both CFS and depression to a group with depression alone. We found that depression looked different in the two groups. Depressed women with CFS had substantially diminished feelings of guilt or worth-lessness compared with those who had depression alone. Also, CFS patients, even when quite depressed, only rarely think about ending their lives to escape their illness. In other words, patients with depression but not CFS are *more* likely to be suicidal. To me, this means that depression in CFS is different from depression that occurs without the physical symptoms consistent with the diagno-sis of CFS. Backing this up is recent work from the University of Washington indicating that rates of suicide in CFS patients were no different from those of the population in general.

Other experiments suggest yet another difference between depression and CFS. These studies explored the role of serotonin, a brain substance that's involved in mood, pain, and fatigue. In depression, serotonin activity goes down. (Although the experi-menter cannot possibly measure brain serotonin in a living person, it is easy to assay a hormone, prolactin, that is a measure of sero-tonin levels.) When depressed patients are given a substance called tryptophan that releases serotonin from certain brain neurons, prolactin is released, but in lower amounts than in healthy people. When CFS patients—regardless of whether they are depressed—participate in this experiment, levels increase but now to values *higher* than found in healthy people. This is the opposite of what occurs in depression.

What do these studies tell us? First, that CFS and depression are probably not the same illness. But they tell us a second thing too. If all depression were the same, then CFS patients with depression should have the same brain chemistry as people with depression alone, and this is not the case. This means that all depression is not the same. Like CFS and FM, depression itself is a syndrome and may have many different causes. Therefore, having the diagnosis of depression in the face of major problems with fatigue or pain may not be the same as having the diagnosis of depression without these symptoms. Psychiatrists usually view the combination of depression with medically unexplained symptoms as just a variant of depression. To me, this is an oversimplification at best. A depressed mood may be the common denominator in both condi-tions, but the variances suggest different underlying brain-related causes and perhaps treatments. Unfortunately, this is an idea that has not yet come of age in psychiatry.

One of the few upsides to depression is that it may cause patients with illnesses like FM to seek medical care. Whenever I diagnose depression in one of my patients, I explain that having depression on top of CFS, FM, or IBS is like turning up the stove under a pot: everything gets hotter. The symptoms of fatigue and pain increase, while the patient's ability to cope with them in the face of other daily demands decreases. So an important component of my evaluation is to consider the possibility of depression.

But what about the much more common case when you feel sad but your symptoms, fortunately, don't add up to a diagnosis of depression? This would be the case if you felt pretty well one week and then sad with frequent crying spells the next. The next step is to try to get a handle on just how depressed you feel. To do this, you should use the standardized questionnaire released by the Center for Epidemiological Studies on Depression (CES-D), which I have reproduced on the next page. It is also available on the Internet with automatic scoring at www.chcr.brown.edu/pcoc/ cesdscale.pdf.

The minimum score at which depression becomes likely in an otherwise well person is 16, but it is 26 for people with medical illness. Scores in the teens are very common in medically unexplained illness and really don't mean clinical depression. However, scores in the 20s catch my attention, while scores in the 30s or 40s definitely concern me. Maybe it is because I am not a psychiatrist, but I think the score on the CES-D is every bit as important as the textbook diagnosis of depression in deciding whether to treat a patient for depression. So if you are quite sad and tearful with a tendency to do less than usual but have occasional good moments, you wouldn't be diagnosed with depression. However, because your depressed mood can still alter your quality of life to a great degree, it should be treated nonetheless.

Research indicates that a rather large number of women with FM don't even bother going to the doctor. They might have gone once or twice in the past, but after they were told there was "nothing wrong," they turn to things they can try themselves, usually

### Depression Screening Form

Rate each statement for how often you felt or behaved this way during the past week. Use the following scale:

0 = Rarely or none of the time (less than one day)
1 = Some or little of the time (one or two days)
2 = Occasionally or a moderate amount of time (three or four days)
3 = Most of the time (five to seven days)

1. I was bothered by things that usually don't bother me.
2. I did not feel like eating; my appetite was poor.
3. I felt that I cold not shake off the blues even with help from my family.
4. I felt that I was just as good as other people.
5. I had trouble keeping my mind on what I was doing.
6. I felt depressed.
7. I felt that everything I did was an effort.
8. I felt hopeful about the future.
9. I thought my life has been a failure.
10. I felt fearful.
11. My sleep was restless.
12. I was happy.
13. I talked less than usual.
14. I felt lonely.
15. People were unfriendly.
16. I enjoyed life.
17. I had crying spells.
18. I felt sad.
19. I felt that people disliked me.
20. I could not get going.

Scoring: For questions 4, 8, 12, and 16, score 3 as 0, 2 as 1, and 1 as 2. For all others questions your response is your score.

Source: Centers for Epidemiological Studies on Depression (CES-D)

ibuprofen and massage. These "nonpatients" have a lower rate of depression than patients who actually seek care. However, not going to the doctor did not protect these people from depression. The simple fact is that people who consult doctors for medical problems have higher rates of depression and other psychiatric problems than people who go it alone. This probably has to do with the fact that people who seek health care tend to be sicker than those who do not.

My colleague Karen Raphael has been studying the relationship between depression and FM by randomly telephoning households where women are present. If a woman Karen calls indicates that she has pain, and that her pain fits the definition of "widespread," Karen asks her to come to our medical school for an evaluation. She asks some of the woman's blood relatives to come in, too, and compares rates of depression in the woman with pain to that in her relatives.

Karen's results have been surprising. First, rates of depression in relatives of women who had neither FM nor depression were 30 percent. This underlines the fact that major depressive disorder is a critical health problem for otherwise healthy women in the twenty-first century. Making this point is another reason this chapter is so important. Second, having a relative who had FM was an added risk factor for having depression. In fact, those relatives had rates of depression equal to rates in relatives of depressed people—a third higher than in those with neither FM nor depression. This finding suggests fibromyalgia and depression share some common familial or genetic denominator, which may be the neurotransmitter serotonin. There will be more information about this substance later in the book.

## Physical Symptoms and Depression

The study of relationships between depression and unexplained medical symptoms has led to additional research that focuses on the unexplained medical conditions themselves. These symptoms, it turns out, account for the lion's share of cases doctors see. One study of 1,000 general medical outpatients identified the fourteen most common body symptoms and found that only 16 percent had a known medical cause, and yet medical students—the well-meaning people who will be tomorrow's doctors—spend their four years of medical school focusing on this 16 percent! If they spent a small percentage of those years on the 84 percent of patients whose symptoms have no apparent medical cause, I would not have needed to write this book.

One issue that further muddies the water is that people with depression or anxiety often do not tell their doctor that they are sad or nervous, but instead focus on their physical symptoms. In fact, of 500 patients coming to the doctor with a new medical complaint, half had physical illness alone with no additional psychiatric problem, 20 percent had physical complaints plus pretty obvious underlying psychiatric disorders (but which were not the reason for the patient's visit), and the rest had psychiatric disorders that were the primary reason for the visit or that were consequences of the primary physical illness. In other words, there was a disconnect between patients and doctors. Either the patients did not communicate their emotional distress or the doctors did not pick it up. But emotional distress and symptoms are clearly related. Another study showed that as the number of medical symptoms went up, so too

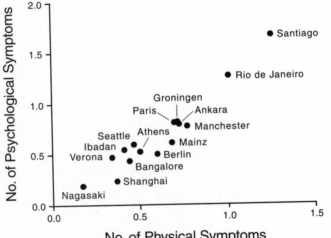

This figure shows the relation between the number of psychological symptoms and the number of physical symptoms in study centers located in fifteen major cities in the world. The relation is considerable and means that as one's burden of symptoms goes up, so do the psychological consequences.

did the risk for major depressive disorder. As to which comes first, that seems to vary from person to person.

The knot between physical symptoms and depression is not limited to the United States, as the graph on page 106 shows. Patients around the world commonly report medical symptoms to their doctors while either ignoring or failing to report symptoms of depression. When asked, most of these people acknowledged that their problems extended to their mood also. Why these people ignore feelings of sadness, hopelessness, and worthlessness to focus on symptoms of fatigue and pain is not clear. My guess has to do with the "tiptoe" quality in the occurrence of depression, which we discussed earlier. Very often, depression comes on so slowly that the person never really notices the change from being a vibrant, alive person to someone shunning human interaction or even going on to have suicidal feelings. In contrast, the threshold for pain or fatigue is a lot narrower. The process producing fatigue, pain, or cognitive dysfunction occurs over a shorter time frame, making it easier to be recognized as abnormal, so the patient goes to the doctor.

Data such as these make it clear that medically unexplained symptoms and major psychiatric disorders such as depression often go hand in hand. For psychiatrists, these studies may seem to indicate that the physical symptoms—pain, fatigue, and others—are nothing more than an extension of the "real" problem: depression. Unable to express the underlying psychiatric disorder, this reasoning goes, the patient creates somatic complaints instead. Psychologists call this unique personality characteristic alexithymia. Unfortunately for this point of view, rates of alexithymia don't differ when patients with medically unexplained symptoms are compared to patients with a medical explanation for their complaints.

My problem with the psychiatric conclusion is that it throws the baby out with the bathwater. It focuses on those cases where medically unexplained symptoms and psychiatric disease do go hand in hand, but these cases never add up to more than 40 percent of the total. Assuming that depression is the "real" disease ignores the majority of cases, where the person with medically unexplained symptoms has no evidence at all of having psychiatric disease.

## Anxiety

Most of us know what anxiety feels like: a feeling of worry or dread that is with us for days, weeks, or months and goes far beyond a normal state of concern. You may experience anxiety when you're under stress, a subject I'll discuss more fully in the next chapter. But here I want to focus on the bodily sensations of anxiety: dry mouth, upset stomach, fatigue, and achy muscles among them. This is another case where the list of symptoms overlaps with symptoms comprising medically unexplained fatigue or pain. I pay particular attention when a patient tells me of feeling anxious or is very stress-sensitive, because these are things that we can treat.

Anxiety is the sister of depression; they often accompany each other, and being depressed is sometimes enough to make people feel anxious. Therefore it is no surprise that treatments for depression often alleviate symptoms of anxiety too. The new class of antidepressants called the selective serotonin reuptake inhibitors, or SSRIs, are particularly good at doing this, and drug companies have found new indications and new populations for this class of drugs. These drugs reverse the tendency for low brain serotonin levels in depression.

An older class of antidepressants, called tricyclic antidepressants, or TCAs, was also effective at reducing anxiety, but general practitioners avoided them due to their frequent and disturbing side effects including an often uncomfortably fast heart rate, weight gain, and very dry mouth. As an alternative to TCAs, practitioners often turned to benzodiazepines, like Valium and Xanax. I very rarely prescribe these drugs because people can become dependent on them. Moreover, the characteristics of these drugs may make it hard to determine whether symptoms are continuing or disappearing. Xanax, for example, melts anxiety away but is very short lived in the body. Because it disappears from the system so quickly, it must be administered at least three times a day. Once Xanax leaves your system, anxiety returns. This raises the question of whether the returning anxiety reflects the underlying problem or is a sign of drug withdrawal. With the patient's other issues, who needs this new problem? Moreover, previous use of a benzodiazepine like Xanax reduces the effect of another drug that's often helpful for anxiety, called Buspar.

## My Own Approach

My private practice is devoted to the care of patients who report major problems with medically unexplained pain or fatigue. Some of these patients show no evidence of depression. Others are depressed but have never been treated for their depression. And a third group is depressed and, by the time they reach me, has had the kitchen sink of drugs thrown at them without any real effect. If you're experiencing pain or fatigue, you undoubtedly fall into one of these three groups, so looking at how I treat each of them might help you understand what you can expect from your own physician.

Unfortunately, when it comes to depression, doctors are less familiar with the science than with their own past experience. This is especially so when it comes time to prescribe drugs. When a pharmaceutical company wants to bring a new antidepressant to market, it must definitively show that its product works better than a placebo, a "sugar" pill that has no biological activity. But the drug company does not have to show that its product works better than products already in the market. So doctors have to choose from among many products, but receive surprisingly little information that helps them make their choices. Doctors tend to try new medicines when they are looking for options beyond their usual ones. Prozac was the first of the new, "cleaner" antidepressants to be released, meaning that patients taking this drug have fewer side effects than patients taking the antidepressants that were previously available. Those drugs, the tricyclics, certainly did reduce depression and anxiety, but at a cost: dry mouth, serious weight gain, and sexual difficulties topping the list.

After Prozac, a wealth of antidepressants hit the market, some of which worked similarly to and some differently from Prozac. So if a doctor was treating a person with depression and Prozac was not effective in reducing the symptoms, he or she might switch to an antidepressant with a different brain action. Unfortunately however, the doctor would be basing the decision on "gut" instinct; the medical literature offers almost no studies that direct doctors on when to make this switch. But literature does exist to make the point that a patient with depression can respond to antidepressant number two when he or she did not respond to antidepressant number one.

So what do I do? That is wholly dependent on the patient. Mine is a "tertiary-care" practice, meaning that I see patients who have already seen their primary-care provider and then at least one specialist. Usually by the time a patient finds me, he or she has seen a dozen doctors. (I guess that means that my practice is "tertiary plus"!) Each of these doctors has probably tried the obvious solutions, including drugs, for the various medically unexplained symptoms the patient exhibits. And since many doctors write off patients complaining of chronic fatigue or pain as being depressed, my new patients are likely to have been given antidepressants by the time they reach me—whether or not they were really depressed. Some patients—those with occult depression—were probably helped, but this shotgun approach, without consideration of underlying depression, is a bad one.

One way to help your doctor help you is to finish this chapter and decide if depression is an issue for you. If so, you can convey this information to your physician and expect to feel better with treatment. If you believe you're not depressed, however, and your physician still suggests antidepressants, you can offer reasons why you suspect this treatment isn't necessary. Since doctors have so much trouble recognizing and treating depression, they need more input from you, the patient, than they routinely get. This kind of active collaboration between you and your doctor will lead to better care. But remember that depression is the "tiptoe" illness. It can come on so slowly that you may be totally unaware that it is there. So if your doctor suspects it, he or she may be right, and a trial of antidepressant medicine might be in order.

Getting the depression diagnosis right is important, since some general practitioners—not just psychiatrists—may turn to antidepressants whenever they're faced with medically unexplained symptoms. They may truly believe you're depressed, or they may simply feel desperate to help. But while certain antidepressants do seem to help with pain (I will discuss this in detail in chapter 7), I find they do little to help patients with severe fatigue who are otherwise in good spirits. In addition, antidepressants, like any other class of drug, have side effects and can be quite expensive. So risk plus cost plus my own experience with their lack of effect for fatigue make it highly unlikely that I'll follow the path of the general practitioner.

Instead, I confine treatment with antidepressants to patients with real depression. Why do I even think about using these drugs when another doctor has already tried them? I reason that if doctors have trouble recognizing depression, they probably don't treat it well. My first step in treating depression, as with any other symptom I treat, is to try to get on the same page as the patient, by asking lots of questions and listening to the answers. Does the patient think depression may be playing a role in the severity of other symptoms and in the ability to deal with them? Very often, the patient says yes but then may become defensive because I've asked about depression when the patient is most concerned about fatigue and pain. This is understandable because doctors in the past said the problem was "all in the head." The patient may tell me that depression is no surprise since life has been so drastically affected by illness. I explain that the hows and whys of having depression do not matter to me. My position is that depression is bad, and its presence makes all other symptoms worse. I also tell the patient that the available treatments are very good at relieving depressive symptoms and only fair in relieving problems with fatigue or pain. With sufficient time to deal with the patient's concerns, this approach usually gets us on the same page in preparation for a trial of medicine to relieve depression.

When Prozac was the only new-generation antidepressant, it was all I used. Now, with more than a dozen new antidepressants available, I rarely use Prozac because it stays in the system for prolonged periods of time. This lingering presence can be a problem when I want to prescribe other drugs, which might interact with Prozac that's still present in the body. So I start with different drugs that are in the same category: SSRIs. I mentioned them before as a treatment for anxiety, but they originally were designed for use in depression. The primary way SSRIs are thought to work is by increasing the amount of serotonin available to parts of the brain that are not receiving enough of this brain-active chemical. The success of this class of drugs in treating depression supports the underlying assumption responsible for their existence: that a lack of serotonin produces the symptoms of depression. However, brain-active chemicals besides serotonin can also affect mood. Altering levels of a different neurotransmitter called norepinephrine (also called noradrenaline) can also alter mood.

When someone with medical symptoms other than pain also has depression, I usually start with drugs in the SSRI class, such as escitalopram (Lexapro). An added benefit of this particular SSRI is that it can also relieve anxiety and sometimes improve sleep. When widespread pain and depression coexist, I choose to prescribe duloxetine (Cymbalta), a drug that alters both serotonin and norepinephrine. I will discuss Cymbalta further when I talk about how I manage severe nonmalignant pain in chapter 7.

The nice thing about using Lexapro is that the starting dose (10 mg) is very often the active dose. If depression remains, it's only one step to the maximum suggested dose of 20 mg. If the depression is unchanged, I will taper off this drug and then, midway through doing this, I will start a drug from a different class, such as Cymbalta or Wellbutrin. If the Lexapro has improved mood in part, I will consider adding a second antidepressant. However, treating depressive symptoms with more than one medicine is often something a primary-care physician is uncomfortable in doing. In my own practice, I often send such patients to a psychiatrist expert in the use of brain-active drugs for help in treating depression. Patients with depression that is resistant to antidepressants—as many as a third of all depressed patients—should be under the care of a psychiatrist.

Many of my patients with both depression and medically unexplained symptoms report having tried many antidepressants with no real benefit. But when I ask about dosages, the patient can rarely remember. So I have to decide whether the patient received an adequate trial of these medicines. Obviously, if the dosage was not sufficient, an ineffective result is not a surprise. So if the patient is willing to try again under my direction, I will simply go through the same protocol as above.

# Monoamine Oxidase Inhibitors (MAOIs)

One well-known class of antidepressants that is not often used nowadays is the monoamine oxidase inhibitors (MAOIs). They're not the easiest drugs for doctors to use, but can be helpful for some patients. MAOIs work very differently from the SSRIs we just discussed. Whereas SSRIs work to increase the availability of the neurotransmitter serotonin, MAOIs work to increase the availability of the other brain-active neurotransmitter involved in regulating mood, norepinephrine. Drugs in either class may be effective in treating depression because the brain cells that release norepinephrine alter the function of the brain cells that release serotonin and vice versa. To say the brain is complicated is certainly an understatement.

MAOIs are thought to be especially useful in treating *atypical* depression, a group of symptoms associated with depression that are just the *opposite* of those seen in typical depression. (Actually "atypical" is probably not a good word to describe these symptoms, because population studies suggest that nearly a third of depressed patients—especially women—have this form of depression.) Where people with typical depression have a sustained depressed mood, those with atypical depression can cheer up in happy situations, only to have the symptoms return again later. And unlike people with ordinary depression, who are likely to lose sleep as well as weight, patients with atypical depression tend to sleep excessively and gain weight, and some may even experience a kind of torpor called *leaden paralysis*. But recall that fluctuating mood, weight gain, excessive sleep, and torpor also describe some patients with severe fatigue. No one has really tested the idea that CFS may in fact be atypical depression. Lacking such a trial, though, I will turn to MAOIs if I am caring for a patient with severe fatigue who also has depression, and who has not responded to other treatments for depression.

As I mentioned, MAOIs are not without risks, although the pharmaceutical industry is currently developing less risky ones. Patients cannot start taking MAOIs until any SSRIs they've taken previously are completely out of their system. They must also watch their diet and avoid certain over-the-counter medicines (see the table on the next two pages). Eating smoked foods, some aged cheeses, and certain other foods while taking the full dosage of an MAOI can be life-threatening, because this mixture can cause your blood pressure to go very high. Obviously, when I explain this to someone who has unsuccessfully tried many other antidepressants, the person is leery of trying this type of drug. Based on the similarity between atypical depression and CFS with depression, however, MAOIs can be worth trying in certain cases—as long as the patient is in the hands of a psychiatrist with experience in using this class of drugs. MAOIs that lack these dietary risks are currently available in Canada and Europe and hopefully will become available in the United States soon. When that happens, I will probably use those drugs as my first line of treatment for depression accompanied by physical symptoms. There will be more to say about a newly available MAOI, administered as a skin patch, in chapter 7.

## Instructions for Patients on MAO Inhibitors

Follow these instructions all the time while taking an MAOI and for two weeks after stopping the drug.

| Foods and Medications | Must Avoid | Allowable |
| --- | --- | --- |
| Dairy Products | Aged cheeses (e.g., blue, Swiss, Cheddar) Homemade yogurt | Unaged cheeses (e.g., cottage, cream, farmer) Yogurt made by reliable manufacturers |
| Alcohol | Red wine Red wine vinegar Rosé Beer Food marinated in beer or wine | White wine Distilled alcohol (alcohol tolerance may be reduced) |
| Fish, meat, poultry | Preserved fish, meat, or poultry (e.g., smoked fish or meat, sausage, salami, pickled herring) | Fresh fish, meat, or poultry Poultry that was fresh when canned or frozen |

| Foods and Medications | Must Avoid | Allowable |
|---|---|---|
| Vegetables | Broad beans (e.g., Chinese snow peas, fava beans, English beans, Italian beans, black beans) | Other legumes and vegetables, including pickled vegetables |
| Fruits | Overripe bananas, banana flavorings<br>Overripe avocados | Firm bananas or avocados<br>Other fruits |
| Beverages | Excessive amounts of caffeinated coffee, tea, cola (more than two cups/cans daily)<br>Marmite, Bovril (beef extracts used in Britain)<br>Excessive amounts of chocolate<br>Excessive amounts of soy sauce | Noncaffeinated beverages |
| Medications | Cough, cold, hay fever, diarrhea preparations (e.g., Contac, Dristan, Sudafed, Acufed, Demerol, Lomotil)<br>Diet pills<br>Amphetamine, cocaine | Antibiotics, hormones aspirin acetaminophen |

# Talk Therapy for Depression and Anxiety

Before the pharmaceutical industry developed the first of what is now a long line of drugs that treat depression and anxiety, the only way to help a patient suffering from these problems was with psychotherapy, a process in which a patient and a professional talk through the problems in the patient's life.

The history of psychotherapy (and especially of its most intensive, expensive form, psychoanalysis) makes the average layperson question its value. But methods for helping people deal with abnormal feeling states have evolved a great deal in the past few decades. Instead of asking someone to discuss his or her dreams or early childhood experiences in excruciating detail, therapists now concentrate on the here and now. A remarkable psychiatrist, Aaron Beck, and an equally remarkable psychologist, Albert Ellis, arrived at a new form of talk therapy called cognitive-behavioral therapy, or CBT. In 2006, Beck was awarded the Albert Lasker Clinical Medical Research Award for his insightful work; this award is often a step to a Nobel prize. Both Beck and Ellis have written books for the layperson that are well worth reading. In contrast to psychoanalysis, CBT has an endpoint: improved daily function for depressed and anxious people. By simply recognizing that his or her beliefs may be contributing to depression, a patient may find the depression beginning to fade, or at least becoming easier to deal with. CBT has helped doctors and patients wipe out depression for some, reduce its symptoms for others, and better understand and cope with what remains for many. Equally important, CBT is not interminable; usually a skilled therapist can help a person get around a depressed mood or anxiety in ten to twelve sessions.

One way to get a better sense of CBT is to turn to the Internet. The National Association of Cognitive Behavior Therapists Web site or that of the Academy of Cognitive Therapy lays out the details of CBT and also provides names of licensed therapists who follow the tenets of the doctors who developed CBT as an effective, highly focused therapy. Another Web-based alternative uses a parallel method developed by Dr. Abraham Low, a neurologist-psychiatrist who lived in the middle of the last century. Dr. Low's system was developed to help patients with conditions such as depression and anxiety learn new ways to reduce their symptoms by talking with people whose symptoms are similar. Currently, more than seven hundred self-help groups using the Low method exist across the country. The Web address is www.recovery-inc.org. The wonderful thing about Recovery Inc. is that it is essentially free, and made up of ordinary people who want to help themselves and others.

Current thinking in psychiatry is that the best way to treat depression or anxiety is with a combination of one of the new antidepressants and CBT. Fifty-five percent of patients with depression showed improvement when they tried with an SSRI alone; 52 percent got better with CBT alone; but 85 percent showed improvement when both treatments were used. In the same way that CBT improves treatment of depression with antidepressants, I strongly believe that

CBT improves treatment of medically unexplained pain and fatigue.

I will discuss in more detail a simple version of CBT in chapter 8 because it is extremely useful in helping people cope with chronic illness, even in the absence of depression. If the chronic illness is depression or anxiety, CBT helps give you perspective on the processes that lead to sadness or being upset. If the sickness is CFS, FM, or IBS, CBT helps you gain a sense of control over your illness. Learning about CBT is as important to a doctor as learning how to use a stethoscope.

To sum up, if depression is present, it's important to whack it with the medical hammer. If the depression lifts with medicines alone, I don't initiate any other treatment. Some patients surprise me by complaining that they have to take medicine. I tell them to think about their depression as if it were diabetes. Both are bad diseases that can be managed with medications. Receiving a prescription from your doctor doesn't necessarily mean you'll be treating your depression with drugs for the rest of your life. Depression is a chronic illness, but one that can disappear completely for short or long periods. When people are concerned about having to take antidepressants for long periods of time, I tell them we'll review the situation in six months. At that point, some people with depression can indeed come off medication, while others may start feeling depressed again. Both treatment and its interruption must be tailored to the individual.

When medicine is helpful but symptoms of depression remain, I send the person to a therapist for CBT. Having CBT available as a backup increases the probability that depression will lift. That alone is wonderful, but there is a second benefit: removing depression turns the heat down on the medical symptoms. The symptoms become less intense, and the sufferer can cope better, because when the physical symptoms decrease, very often the psychological ones do also. So CBT offers a two-way street. Less depression may produce less of a problem with symptoms. That in turn may resolve the depression completely.

Now let's turn our attention to issues that interfere with wellness and, in and of themselves, can produce fatigue and pain—namely, stress and sleep.

# 6

# Step Two: Removing Stress and Improving Sleep

As you now understand, depression can produce symptoms of fatigue and achiness on its own, making any medical illness worse. Fortunately, it can be treated. Stress is similarly two-headed. If you're in good physical health but under substantial emotional or mental stress, you will not feel well, because stress produces symptoms. And if you have another illness—including severe fatigue or pain—stress will make it worse. In fact, recent work has suggested that stress is a risk factor for the later development of medically unexplained fatigue.

What is stress and why am I discussing it here? First, stress is your body's response to things in the environment that are emotionally arousing. These environmental stimuli are called stressors. Very often, stressors are annoying or negative experiences—like having to take an exam, having your job performance evaluated by a superior, or arguing with a family member. But sometimes the environmental stimulus is positive—like getting married or going to an exciting movie. Obviously what produces stress varies from person to person; or, if you will, one person's stressor is another person's pleasure. Stress is important because if you are stressed out, all your symptoms will get worse. So stress, like depression, is a symptom multiplier. Moreover, stress occurring earlier in life is a risk factor for developing chronic fatigue.

# Stress Plus Unexplained Illness

You know already that medically unexplained illnesses stem from physical causes, yet recovery may involve dealing with emotional and psychological symptoms. In the last chapter, we noted that focusing *only* on the physical causes of your illness may, in fact, slow your recovery. It's important to address the physical issues, but as long as you're dealing only with pain and fatigue you will probably feel that you have less control over your recovery. In order to get on the path to wellness, it's important to step back from your illness and look deeper within yourself at elements that might be slowing your recovery.

Stress is the number one overlooked factor on the path to wellness. Mental stress, like physical exertion, can make symptoms worse. Here's an extreme example: Do you recall Hurricane Andrew, the devastating storm that struck Florida in 1992? Chronic fatigue syndrome (CFS) patients who lived through that terrible disaster reported significant worsening of all their symptoms. It's no surprise that living through a major hurricane would be a stressful experience, but why should this event have been especially difficult for CFS patients? The reasons start with the body's immune system.

Invasion of the body by foreign pathogens is the process that usually sets the immune system going. The pathogen is detected in the blood by immune active cells that turn on the manufacture of chemicals called *cytokines*. And the release of cytokines, in turn, produces fatigue, achiness, and cognitive dysfunction—one reason why you might feel tired or a little disoriented while fighting a cold or the flu, even at times when you're otherwise in good health. But your body can also release cytokines when you're under stress. The researchers studying the CFS patients caught in the hurricane thought that stress-related cytokine release had made the patients more sick. Stopping stress, not surprisingly, dampens immune system activity, thus reducing levels of cytokines. So removing stress from your life prevents the added dose of fatigue on top of your existing symptoms.

You may have no stress in your life other than your illness, or you may have additional stressors. Even if your life is an ocean of calm other than your illness, however, the pain or fatigue you're already fighting is certainly a gargantuan stressor. Even if there are really no other significant stresses in your life, it's still important to deal with the stress that your illness may be causing you. Doing so will help you reduce the symptoms you're already experiencing. In this chapter, I'll explain the whats and hows of stress and some ways to reduce it and its biological consequences. Whether it is your reaction to your illness or problems with your spouse, child, work, or something else, ignoring the role of stress in inhibiting wellness leads to continued illness. Coping with stress is part of my path to wellness.

## Stress Produces Symptoms

Stress, like depression, is an illness mimicker as well as an illness producer. Take Carol Day, for example. Ms. Day, a thirty-four-year-old single mother, was working three jobs as a personal trainer and yoga instructor. Her jobs were not close by, resulting in a lot of commuting. Moreover, whenever Ms. Day led a class, she would push herself harder than the class itself—more weights, more repetitions. And her child was four years old, with plenty of energy, not to mention all the usual childhood infections. Ms. Day felt she had to do more but in less time—she was a modern supermom.

Ms. Day started to develop vague symptoms of fatigue accompanied by headache and constant muscle soreness, but she kept on going. Finally, she melted down and found herself unable to get out of bed. She had stress-induced exhaustion made worse by the physical demands of her jobs. In essence, she was overtraining—working out more than her body could handle. Overtraining is a particular problem for some elite athletes. To deal with her problem, she completely stopped exercising and went on sick leave for five weeks. Then, she slowly returned to her former life—but far more aware that the circumstances in her life had precipitated this rather long bout of severe fatigue.

You don't have to be an athlete to develop stress-related fatigue. Sedentary, nonathletic people often feel exhausted when under stress. Stress causes anxiety, anxiety disturbs sleep, and then fatigue results. When Ms. Day cut back on all her activities and began to look at her life, she saw that she was burning the candle at both ends. Being removed from the workplace for five weeks gave her time to rest and to rethink some of her strategies of living—and then change them. This woman was unusual in that she figured it out for herself. She might have gone to the doctor to hear there was nothing wrong with her. What would have happened to her if she did not take a time-out from her hectic life? Who knows? But stress is something to be taken very seriously. Therefore, you should understand some of the basic facts and biology of stress.

## What Is Stress?

One person's stress is another's satisfaction, so there really is no way to guess what will cause a stress reaction in any one person. Lots of factors may determine what kinds of events will cause you stress; some may be genetic, while others may have to do with specific kinds of situations. And different people will try to cope with stress in different ways. I define stress as behavioral and biological reactions to some disturbance in your personal environment. What I mean by "disturbance in the environment" is pretty general. It can range from an unexpected torrential rain when you're without your umbrella to being forced into a basement when a once-in-a-lifetime hurricane goes past. But emotional "disturbances" in the environment can trigger stress too: a nasty boss, an argument with a spouse, a problem with a child or an aging parent. There really are a million different stressors, and each is specific to the person.

## The Behavioral Index of Stress

Stressed people tend to be restless and anxious, but these visible signs aren't the end of the story, merely clues to what we're feeling inside. Some people can appear restless and anxious but be quite calm inside. Others may feel anxiety rising within them yet suppress their physical reactions to it; they don't *seem* nervous or stressed, but the story may be very different inside their bodies. If you are the kind of person who actually exhibits the symptoms of stress on the outside—maybe through trembling, or nervous glances around you—then your recognition of these physical reactions can be a very useful way for you to understand when you're under stress. But some people may not be aware they're stressed at all, even though stress may already be doing physical damage to them inside. Only later may biological symptoms begin to emerge.

*Biological* means that the nerves that connect the brain to the various organs of the body begin actively firing. Often when this happens, one of the first physical signs will be problems with sleep. In order for us to get a good night's sleep, we must be able to relax until the processes that control sleep take over. A stressed person can be exhausted during the daytime but suddenly feel revved up at night. Lying in bed, eyes closed, thinking about problems does not allow for the kind of restful state required for a person to transition from wakefulness to sleep. Frequent awakenings are a similar problem. If you can remember becoming awake more than three times in a night, your sleep was probably very disturbed. These patterns of sleep disturbance are quite different from what happens in depression; there, you may fall asleep easily and not wake up during the night, only to wake up extremely early in the morning. In the case of stress, you'll have trouble getting to sleep in the first place, or wake up frequently once you finally drift off.

What are some markers for stress, beyond a disruption of your sleep habits? A common one is muscle tension—extreme tightness in the jaw muscles or in the muscles supporting the head. Muscle contraction can be excruciating and can lead to what you may perceive as a headache (actually a neck ache so severe that the pain spreads up across your head) or pain on opening or closing the mouth. When I examine such a patient, her jaw, neck, and upper shoulder muscles will usually be extremely tender. If you were this patient and told your dentist about your jaw pain, he might make the diagnosis of temporomandibular disorder (TMD). But that is not the correct diagnosis. You're actually suffering a stress-related muscle spasm, albeit severe. Reduce the stress and the pain will go away.

A whole range of stress symptoms stems from the activation of your autonomic nervous system (ANS), which connects your brain to your heart, stomach, salivary glands—essentially all the organs within the body cavities. As soon as your brain senses stress, the autonomic nerves alter their firing rates with consequences that you can feel—a faster heart rate, rumbling in the stomach, sudden dry mouth. There's a very good reason for your body to behave this way. Your brain interprets stress in the same way it interprets emergencies or bodily threats. It creates this "fight or flight" response because it wants to prepare you to do just that: fight some attacker like a wild animal or flee from it. But in the modern world, we're less likely to encounter these primitive threats than we are to encounter a surly boss, a traffic jam, or a bumpy airline flight—all events that might trigger the same response of your ANS. Tensing your muscles or increasing your heart rate serves no real purpose in these contemporary situations, but they can make you feel physically or emotionally stressed, or both. And if you have these physical reactions often enough, you will become achy and fatigued.

One important fact to take away from this discussion, no matter what the origin of your stress, is that it's important to recognize its signs. If you find yourself waking up repeatedly during the night for no reason, or leaving work early because of tight neck muscles that have caused a miserable headache, you may simply be dealing with the natural responses to some difficult situation. Regardless, it's important to think about the reasons so that you can begin to eliminate them. This is especially important when you're also trying to cope with medically unexplained illnesses, which add their own stresses to your life.

## What to Do about Stress

There are three major ways of dealing with stress. One is to ignore it until it becomes so debilitating that your health suffers. Assuming you see why this isn't a good alternative, you can use either self-help or professional help to get to the bottom of your stress and begin eliminating it. Several self-help techniques will seem obvious as I describe them, but surprisingly often they're anything but obvious to an individual who's under stress. One of them is taking time off from the problems and issues that are causing the stress in the first place. When I encounter a patient with medically unexplained symptoms and a load of stress in her life, the first question I ask is when the person last had a vacation. If it has been more than a year, I take out my prescription pad and write VACATION. At a minimum, I prescribe four days away from the usual surroundings and their attendant stresses. Four days isn't much time, but it may be long enough to prove that the "usual" situation isn't helping her health.

Because stress is so much a part of the life of the average American, stress management has become a cottage industry in the United States. There are plenty of books, Web sites and experts to help you manage your stress load. My goal in this chapter is not to replace them. That would require an entire book (and probably a change of career for me). Instead, what I want to do is to give you an overview of the methods modern psychology has developed to help you manage stress.

## Exercise

A major tool to use against stress is physical exercise. Exercise relieves stress by turning down the ANS and putting it into your control. The symptoms of increased ANS activity that we've already discussed—an accelerated heart rate, dry mouth, stomach cramps, muscle spasms, and more—are uncomfortable when you're not exercising. But when you exercise, these changes have a purpose—namely to shift blood flow from your mouth and gut to your muscles. You may not be running from a wild animal, but you're channeling blood—and the oxygen it carries—to the muscles you're using to run, bike, lift weights, or whatever exercise you've chosen. The more blood is sent to the muscles, the more oxygen is delivered, resulting in longer and higher performance exercise. So when you exercise, autonomic activation is not uncomfortable. Moreover, as you exercise at higher intensities, the ANS's response to exercise shifts down a gear. Your nervous system becomes used to the kinds of activities that exercise involves, and doesn't feel compelled to shift you into "fight or flight" mode every time some petty annoyance (like a traffic jam) gets in your way. A regular exerciser is, in fact, less stress responsive biologically than a sedentary person. This means less dry mouth and a slower heart rate, or, if you will, less stress.

The problem, of course, is the requirement to exercise. Most of us talk about how we should be exercising, but far fewer Americans really make regular exercise a priority. But if you identify stress as a problem for you, you really have far more reason—and incentive—to use exercise. Don't worry too much about overtraining, the problem Carol Day experienced; for most of us, the problem is undertraining or not training at all. You may find exercise incredibly rewarding—even addicting—and, in contrast to drugs, the side effects are unusually benign. Exercise combats stress by tuning down the ANS by releasing endorphins, the body's endogenous opiates. Their release is associated with the well described "runner's high." Although running is not necessary to reduce stress, some form of active, rather vigorous exercise is. There will be an exercise prescription in chapter 8.

## Other Ways to Manage Stress

Walking, yoga, and tai chi are an integral part of the gentle physical conditioning program in chapter 8, so be sure to look at that later chapter. Beyond these physical programs, it's worth discussing imaging, progressive muscular relaxation, and the Relaxation Response, all common methods of reducing stress that are easy and enjoyable. In imaging, you listen to a tape (often available at your local library) and concentrate on putting yourself in the situation portrayed on the tape. Usually, you're asked to picture yourself in a very pleasant environment and then to focus on that environment, freeing your mind of distracting thoughts. In progressive muscular relaxation, you're asked to activate specific muscle groups as much as you possibly can and then suddenly let loose. This process allows you to relax muscles that stress has tightened. Usually you start with the hands, contract them maximally for a count of five, then gently but quickly relax while exhaling. You move from the hands to the lower arms, the upper arms, shoulders, and so on. Neck and shoulder relaxation are probably the most helpful as these combat the muscle tension that leads to headache. The tape will instruct you to go through muscle groups beginning with your hands and ending in your face. By the time you are finished, you have essentially given yourself a physical workout—albeit without running—and you will feel less stressed.

Meditation is an excellent stress management tool, but many

Americans have problems with the requirement to chant specific formulaic mantras and to deal with non-Western concepts like the "third eye." The Relaxation Response was developed by Harvard's Dr. Herbert Benson as a means of demystifying meditation and making it easy for everyone to do. Specific instructions can be found at several Web sites (for example, see www.ucop.edu/humres/eap/relaxationrespone.html). Essentially all you have to do is sit in a quiet place with your eyes closed. Then concentrate on relaxing all your muscles—starting at your toes and moving up toward your head. Then breathe easily and naturally through your nose and as you end each breath, say "One." Do this for ten to twenty minutes per day. As you meditate in this way, your mind might wander; just bring your attention back to your breathing. You'll find that the Relaxation Response is even easier to induce following physical exertion, so if you're able to use both, you should see an especially significant dent in your stress levels.

For people who have problems getting into this form of self-meditation, there's a device available called the resperate that makes this easy. Go to www.resperate.com to check it out. The resperate has actually been approved for the treatment of high blood pressure, which, in part, is due to high activity of the ANS, which connects the brain to all the hollow organs of the body including the blood vessels. The device works to lower high blood pressure by tuning down the ANS by helping you to learn how to breathe as if you were doing the Relaxation Response. With this device, all you have to do is breathe in when the tone goes up in pitch and breath out when the tone goes down in pitch. Very gradually these tones help you slow your breathing and stretch it out into a pattern that relieves stress. The downside to any device, of course, is that there is a cost involved. If that is not a major impediment, it really is worth trying. It is not boring and you will find it very relaxing. It is a very good way of managing stress.

### Turning to a Therapist

Helping people deal with stress is the bread and butter of clinical psychology in the twenty-first century. A major technique psychologists use for this purpose is biofeedback. In biofeedback, the therapist is the middleman between you, your physiology, and a computer that can detect stress. Once the therapist has a better sense of what's causing your body to react to stress, he or she can teach you ways to turn off your stress responses. However, with advances in computerization, the middleman may no longer be necessary. Biofeedback will appear in more detail in chapter 8 as a method that concentrates on reducing stress by improving breathing. In that chapter, you will find a way to do it yourself.

Although you can take a vacation without help and you can give yourself biofeedback without help, you may nonetheless want a professional to help you manage your stress load. Good for you. You've recognized that stress really is a contributor to your pain or fatigue (or both) and you've also realized you may have a tough time overcoming it yourself. I would recommend professional psychological help, however, in one of two conditions. One is if you have problems doing these self-help methods on your own. Don't feel bad; you're not alone. Eighty percent of Americans will be in your boat—the same percentage who have never exercised and cannot easily see themselves exercising now. If self-help were easy, there wouldn't be jobs for psychologists. The second condition is if you're willing, and able, to pay for professional help. Medical insurance reimbursement for psychological services is often abysmal, and psychologists—while often flexible about fees depending on your ability to pay—may not always be inexpensive. On the other hand, stress reduction therapies usually do not take very long and so the cost to you, in both time and money, will not be great. Probably the best way to find a stress management professional will be to ask a friend or relative who has used one in the past; your physician may also have suggestions. Barring that, try typing the words "stress management" and the name of your state and county into a Web search engine. Your search should yield plenty of choices.

## Sleep and Common Causes of Disturbed Sleep

People with medically unexplained fatigue and pain complain bitterly of problems sleeping. These range from problems falling asleep to frequent arousals during the night, to early awakening and a need to sleep many hours but without being refreshed in the morning. The question is whether you have an underlying sleep disorder producing these problems. Such a sleep disorder would provide a medical explanation for your symptoms and would require care by a specialist in sleep medicine.

Recognizing sleep disorders is difficult. Experts in sleep medicine usually ask patients about sleepiness—the inability to stay awake even in situations when wakefulness is required, such as at work or while driving. The Epworth Sleepiness Scale (reproduced on the next page) is commonly used to screen a person for excessive daytime sleepiness. The scale was tested on a large group of healthy people whose scores never exceeded 10, while people with sleep disorders often had higher scores. The operative word is *often*. A score of over 9 is considered sleepy and over 17 is very sleepy. Having a high Epworth score does not necessarily mean that you will have a sleep disorder diagnosed by an overnight sleep study, but the chances are a lot higher than if your Epworth is low. That's why the Epworth should be viewed as a screening test rather than a diagnostic test. The drawback to the Epworth is that it asks you to assess your own sleepiness and so is a subjective measure of sleepiness. A more objective measure brings you into a darkened room during the daytime after a full night of sleep—to see how long it takes for you to fall asleep. The cutoff point for this sleep latency test is eight minutes. If you fall asleep faster than that, you are much sleepier than a normal person, and you probably have a sleep disorder, which could be treatable.

If you score 10 or more on the Epworth test, you should consider whether you are obtaining adequate sleep, need to improve your sleep hygiene, and/or need to see a sleep specialist. These issues should be discussed with your personal physician.

Many people with sleep disorders complain of fatigue but not always of sleepiness. Although fatigue and sleepiness often overlap, they don't have to. For example, many of my CFS patients are extremely fatigued but also have major problems falling asleep. So they are fatigued but not sleepy. Sorting out similarities and differences between fatigue and sleepiness is the subject of a research project I'm currently conducting with Dr. Alexandros Vgontzas, a sleep researcher at Pennsylvania State University medical school.

---

### The Epworth Sleepiness Scale

Use the following scale to choose the number that best represents your chance of dozing or sleeping in each of the situations listed. Write the appropriate number on the blank line next to each situation.

0 = would *never* doze or sleep
1 = *slight* chance of dozing or sleeping
2 = *moderate* chance of dozing or sleeping
3 = *high* chance of dozing or sleeping

1. Sitting and reading                                        _____
2. Watching TV                                                _____
3. Sitting inactive in a public place                        _____
4. Being a passenger in a motor vehicle for an
   hour or more                                               _____
5. Lying down in the afternoon                                _____
6. Sitting and talking to someone                            _____
7. Sitting quietly after lunch (no alcohol)                  _____
8. Stopped for a few minutes in traffic while driving        _____
   Total score                                               _____

---

While it would make sense that people with severe fatigue or widespread pain might have an underlying sleep disorder, the evidence for this possibility is not convincing. While many studies (including my own) find that sleep disorders occur no more often in patients with medically unexplained symptoms than in the general population, one sleep specialist at the medical school in Stony Brook, New York, has reported a mild form of sleep apnea to be common in patients with fibromyalgia (FM). One reason for the apparent discrepancy is that most sleep studies report on small numbers of patients. We are currently collecting sleep data on more and more patients with CFS or FM to evaluate further the idea that some may have sleep disorders causing their symptoms; our preliminary analysis, however, is negative. I do think it is critical that you have a good understanding of the common sleep disorders, and so I will have more to say about them later in this chapter. This will provide you the information needed to discuss the possibility of your having a sleep study with your doctor.

Disturbed sleep can be caused by many factors. We've already talked about how stress can interfere with your ability to fall asleep. Most of us, however, don't get enough sleep because we simply don't make enough time for it, or we set up completely artificial conditions that make it very difficult to get to sleep. Sleep needs to be a priority, especially when you're not feeling well; a lack of sleep will only add to the fatigue you may already be feeling. In addition, sleep deprivation itself can produce diffuse muscular achiness as well as problems with concentration. And people sleep less than they think. One study reported that the average time in bed for a large number of adults was 7.5 hours. However, the actual time asleep averaged 6.7 hours for white women and almost an hour less for black women. This is simply not enough. Estimate your sleep time by the amount of time you are in bed each night. If you have a problem with fatigue and achiness and are sleeping less than seven hours a night, your first goal should be to increase the amount of sleep you're getting. As you get used to having longer sleep durations, over the course of several weeks, you should start feeling more refreshed upon awakening.

One problem that leads to difficulties with sleep is using your bed as your office. Too many people can't bring themselves to turn out the light and get comfortable when they go to bed. Instead they read, watch television, or even start paying their bills. Finally, they may turn out the light and lie down, only to find themselves staring at the ceiling, wide awake. What's happened? They've made being in bed so much like sitting on the sofa, or at a brightly lit desk, that the difference between sitting up and lying down is no longer very great. Using your bed as an office tends to extinguish your body's normal association between bed and sleep, which triggers sleepiness. The link between bed and falling asleep is very much akin to what happens to a dog that learns food will be provided whenever a bell rings. Pretty soon, the sound of a bell will cause the dog to salivate even when there's no food around. Be sure to relearn this good association by reserving your bed for sleeping only.

Other things that interfere with sleep are cigarettes, alcohol, and of course caffeine. A cigarette is a nonpharmacological way of injecting nicotine into your body. Nicotine is a stimulant, and its use can make falling asleep harder for smokers than for nonsmokers. You shouldn't smoke at all, of course, but if you do, make a point of putting your cigarettes away after 7 p.m. The story is the same for alcohol. Alcohol is a sedating drug. Using it will ordinarily put you to sleep; but if you use too much, your sleep will be disturbed. You'll either wake up more frequently or awaken in the morning feeling unrefreshed. Most people will have no problem with one or two glasses of wine (or drinks), but have more than that and you may find sleep a dicey proposition.

Finally there's the issue of caffeine. Everyone knows that the function of caffeine is to wake you up. That is why so much coffee flows in the morning. But caffeine is a drug that stays in your body for at least six hours (and for some people a lot longer than that), so ingesting it late in the day can disturb night sleep. Although most people are well aware that caffeine is in coffee, they sometimes forget that it is also in colas and other soft drinks, many teas, and even chocolate. A nice cup of hot cocoa before bed may seem like a relaxing idea, but it could actually keep you awake for hours. You have to stop drinking caffeinated beverages after one in the afternoon to avoid these negative effects, especially if you are sensitive to caffeine. So if you have trouble sleeping, your first course of action is to stop smoking and stop drinking alcohol and caffeinated drinks.

What should people with medically unexplained fatigue or pain do about smoking, alcohol, and caffeine? They too should stop using these drugs. Besides all its other health risks, nicotine is associated with fatigue. To stop using it is a no brainer. When I ask my patients about alcohol, the vast majority tell me they do not drink except on rare social occasions. If they have a chemical sensitivity, they often report that alcohol gives them an instant headache and horrible malaise, so they tend to stay away from this drug. So for the great bulk of patients who consult with me, alcohol is not an issue. For those who do use it, moderation is critical or else your sleep could be affected. I'll mention caffeine as a treatment for fatigue in the next chapter.

## Sleep Disorders

Sometimes, however, overconsumption of alcohol or caffeine, smoking, or poor bedtime habits simply don't explain why a person can't sleep. When I am faced with someone who reports having major problems with sleep and always feels unrefreshed, I consider the possibility of a sleep disorder. Although the correlation between medically unexplained symptoms and a sleep disorder is not high, it is always a possibility for the individual patient. If I can diagnose a medically known sleep disorder, I can offer treatment for it.

## Narcolepsy

Narcolepsy is rare, occurring about once in 2,000 people (that makes it as common as multiple sclerosis [MS]), and is more common in men than women. Patients with narcolepsy have pathological daytime sleepiness regardless of how well they sleep at night. One moment they are awake, and the next moment unable to stay awake—even while driving a car. The problem is an abnormal sleep system related to a reduction of a brain chemical called *hypocretin*. Sleep study is diagnostic in that patients with narcolepsy fall quickly into rapid eye movement (REM) sleep, an occurrence not seen for an hour or two in people whose sleep is normal. REM sleep never occurs during the daytime in most people but does occur *suddenly* in people with narcolepsy and explains the daytime sleep attacks that occur. Another diagnostic test for narcolepsy is to determine the time to nap during daytime. Very often, the sleep latency is in the order of a few minutes, well below the cutoff of 8 minutes.

The first line of treatment for narcolepsy-induced daytime sleepiness is a drug called modafinil (Provigil). This drug has been available for the treatment of narcolepsy since 1999. Prior to modafinil, the drug treatment most used for sleepiness was a cerebral stimulant, like methylphenidate or amphetamine. These drugs kept patients with narcolepsy awake, but they also produced a host of side effects, including anxiety, muscle tremulousness, trouble sleeping, and headache. I'll have more to say about all these treatments in the next chapter.

The mode of action of modafinil is not known, but it seems to target fatigue without as many side effects as the cerebral stimulants. I say "as many" advisedly. In my experience with using this drug in patients with severe and long-lasting fatigue, about half have such disturbing side effects that they prefer not take the medicine. Nevertheless, modafinil is still the number one medical treatment for narcolepsy. When it fails, the treating doctors try methylphenidate or amphetamine. Finally, doctors suggest that patients try to nap in order to ward off sleep attacks at inopportune times, like when driving or bathing a child.

### Delayed Sleep Phase Disorder

This syndrome has to do with an abnormality of the biological clock. Most people get sleepy at night, sometime between 10 p.m. and 1 a.m. But people with *delayed sleep phase disorder* can't fall asleep before 3 or 4 a.m. or even later. Obviously if you have to be at work at 9 a.m., this is a problem. When I evaluate a patient, I inquire about sleep start and end times as well as about the quality of sleep. Answers outside of the normal range suggest a diagnosis of this disorder.

What to do about it? Here are a few recommendations. People with delayed sleep phase disorder may try going to bed 30 to 60 minutes earlier each week, until they're finally going to bed at a normal time. Doing this allows their biological clock to gradually adjust to falling asleep a bit earlier each week. Another option is exposure to extremely bright light in the morning (10,000 lux fluorescent fixtures) for about 30 minutes. In some cases, a low dose of melatonin several hours before normal bedtime may also be helpful.

### Restless Legs Syndrome

The third disorder is called restless legs syndrome (RLS), and it is common, occurring in about 5 percent of people, with women affected more often than men. Many people have some discomfort in their legs at night but don't report fatigue. To receive this diagnosis, the person has to give the appropriate history plus complain of severe fatigue or marked daytime sleepiness. So in evaluating sleep, I ask patients if their legs are uncomfortable as they are falling asleep, and if wiggling them makes them feel better. If they answer yes, I diagnose RLS. This sensation in their legs is brought on by inactivity—sitting or lying down—and is worse at night.

Individuals with more severe forms of RLS report having involuntary movements of the arms or legs, even while they are awake.

There really is no test that can diagnose RLS, so, in this regard, it resembles some of the other "illnesses" we have discussed so far. But something is known about possible causes. Family factors play an important role, and rates of RLS zoom in frequent blood donors who have an iron deficiency.

How this syndrome is treated depends mostly on how bad it is. But the first thing the doctor will do is check out the body's iron stores by testing ferritin levels. If these are low, he or she is likely to prescribe iron pills. The mainstays of treatment for RLS, though, are also treatments for Parkinson's disease or for epilepsy. Patients with RLS don't have either of these diseases, but the medicines used to treat them also greatly reduce the symptoms of RLS. In fact, the FDA has officially approved several of these drugs for the treatment of moderate to severe RLS. Interestingly, one of them, pramipexole (Mirapex), has also been reported to reduce pain and fatigue in patients with fibromyalgia. This result may lead to additional testing of this class of drugs as a treatment for disturbed sleep with widespread pain.

Although those of my patients who have tried the anti-Parkinson's medicines report improvement, some patients taking these drugs for long periods of time complain that the RLS gets worse: it may start earlier in the day or affect more of the body. When this happens, the doctor may try an antiepileptic drug such as gabapentin (Neurontin) or very low doses of medicines in the codeine class of drugs.

## Sleep-Disturbed Breathing

The last group of sleep disorders is the most common. Sleep-disturbed breathing occurs in up to 20 percent of the population. Its worst form is sleep apnea, an illness primarily of overweight, middle-aged men. Women are, in fact, protected from sleep apnea while they are menstruating. But after the age of fifty, with the loss of the protective reproductive hormones and the resulting gain in weight, rates in women approach those in men.

Sleep apnea is characterized by very loud snoring with occasional periods when the person not only stops snoring, but stops breathing altogether. If you are this person's bedmate, this can be very disturbing. You wonder if your bedmate is going to wake up. Oddly, this means that the sleep apnea patient and his partner may both find themselves experiencing daytime fatigue—one from being awakened repeatedly when his breathing stops, and the other from being kept awake by the spouse's loud snoring—or worry over his total lack of breathing.

Sleep apnea is caused by the combination of sleep-related muscular relaxation and weight-related thickening of the respiratory passages. That's why this condition is seen most often in heavy people with thick necks. When such a person falls asleep, the airway is no longer held open and starts to collapse, and the person begins to snore. When the airway collapses completely, the person continues to try to breathe, but air does not get in. This is "apnea," and it usually results in the patient's waking up. These periods of apnea may also cause the body to receive insufficient oxygen, leading to high blood pressure or even heart disease.

A milder form of sleep-disturbed breathing is called *upper airway resistance syndrome* (UARS). Half of all UARS patients are women, and half of them are premenopausal, and, in contrast to the typical patient with sleep apnea, many UARS patients are not overweight. But the complaints sound very much the same as those of patients with sleep apnea: poor quality of sleep, frequent awakenings, and daytime fatigue or sleepiness. Here the problem is frequent arousals throughout the night and not apnea. The medical consequences of these arousals and mild blockages to breathing are still under investigation. Although they may differ from the consequences of severe apnea, that does not make them insignificant. People with UARS tend to have lower blood pressure and report more problems with feeling faint than people with other sleep disorders.

This correlation and a study that shows the same relationship in reverse may actually end up helping a great many patients with chronic fatigue. People with low blood pressure, it turns out, complain of persistent fatigue more often than those with higher blood pressure, and this relation is strongest in women under fifty. These two studies raise the possibility that women with fatigue and low blood pressure may have a treatable sleep disorder. Moreover, one recent study from the medical school at Stony Brook found higher rates of irritable bowel syndrome (IBS) in patients with UARS than in patients with more severe forms of sleep-disturbed breathing. The Stony Brook researchers believe that UARS could explain some cases of medically unexplained fatigue and pain. In a follow-up study to which I alluded earlier, the researchers found a very high rate of UARS in patients with FM. Furthermore, they reported that treatment of sleep-disturbed breathing in these women with the methods I will discuss next greatly reduced their FM symptoms. This is an important finding, but it is one that my colleagues and I have not found; however, we have focused our studies on CFS. I have recently begun a sleep study which I will discuss more in chapter 7. That study should allow me to confirm (or not) the results of the Stony Brook researchers and to sort out whether sleep pathology occurs in FM but not in CFS.

Since patients with UARS don't necessarily have to snore or to be obese with thick necks, the cause of their problem may not be the same as with sleep apnea. Nonetheless, UARS and sleep apnea are diagnosed the same way: by overnight sleep studies that record the number of apneas, incidents of reduced air flow, and arousals. And the treatment of patients across the full range of sleep-disturbed breathing is the same: methods to overcome the obstruction in the airway during sleep. An easy thing to try is an elasticized bandage strip on the nose; these may help open the nasal passages, which could reduce the milder forms of snoring. Unfortunately, this treatment does not work well enough to treat most patients with significant sleep apnea.

Sometimes the problem can be resolved simply by changing your sleep position. Many snorers stop snoring when they shift from their backs to their sides. But overweight people are more comfortable sleeping on their backs. To teach yourself to sleep on your side, you can try a snore-ball. Sew a pocket onto the back of a T-shirt and insert half a tennis ball into the pocket. When you lie on your back wearing the T-shirt, the snore-ball will feel uncomfortable, causing you to roll over onto your side.

Other treatments require seeing a specialist. The least bothersome is when a dentist who is an expert in helping patients with sleep-disturbed breathing prepares a special bite plate that pulls your tongue forward. The standard treatment, however, is a small pump that keeps the airway open by blowing air through a small mask fitted over your nose. This treatment, called continuous positive airway pressure (CPAP), was used by the Stony Brook group to relieve FM symptoms. Finally, surgery may be used to alter the shape of the soft palate, or even the position of the jaw.

People with frequent awakenings, a great deal of fatigue, and high values on the Epworth Sleepiness Score should talk to their doctors about having an overnight sleep study. Doing this is the first step in diagnosing all of these examples of treatable causes of severe fatigue.

So where are we now? This chapter and the previous one were necessary for those of you with fatigue and pain of relatively recent onset, because problems with masked depression, stress, or sleep could be the culprits. I needed to lay out the facts on these issues for you to sort through and think over. The demands of the twenty-first century make stress a common accompaniment of everyday life. And we all have our own personal stress "breaking point," the point when we feel uncomfortable or even sick while under stress. Individuals with a high breaking point appear to manage stress well, while those with a low breaking point easily melt down. So the stress load is critical. When the load exceeds your particular breaking point, fatigue and pain are common—either due to the stress itself or to its effect on interfering with restorative sleep.

But what if you continue to feel ill despite taking these factors into account? In the next two chapters I lay out my plan for getting on the road to wellness. Chapter 7 explores a pharmacological approach to handling fatigue (not so great) and pain (rather good), while chapter 8 provides an approach whereby you can gain control over your illness. By taking the reins of your illness into your own hands, you become empowered. A positive outlook is powerful medicine. Defeating the sense of helplessness and being a victim of disease is a shift from negativism to positivism. This shift will make you feel better, and feeling better provides you rays of hope— the start of a cycle moving you progressively to wellness.

# 7

# Step Three: The Role of Drugs in Relieving Pain, Fatigue, and Poor Sleep

Just because a doctor does not know the cause of an illness doesn't mean he or she cannot help the patient reduce the severity of the symptoms. Helping people cope with illness-induced symptoms is a major part of what physicians do. Surgeons, not physicians, cure many diseases by physically removing them from the body, but that's an act that, no matter how much sophistication it requires, still seems primitive to me. In contrast, physicians match symptom, syndrome, or disease with the myriad possibilities in the modern drug pharmacopeia with the goal of improving health and quality of life. Learning how to do this highly sophisticated matching is a major reason why physicians have to go to medical school.

The operative words here are "improve health." Despite all its advances, modern medicine can only cure vitamin deficiencies, bacterial infections and a few caused by viruses, and the rare cancer. We still can't cure viruses that range from the common cold to the ones causing SARS or HIV. But while most medicines are not curative, they certainly can help the patient, either by beating back the cause of the disease or by reducing symptoms. The new medicines for HIV disease are illustrative. The human immunodeficiency virus (HIV) causes acquired immune deficiency syndrome (AIDS). If this virus is left untreated, more than 90 percent of the people it infects will die. The virus grows and grows, eventually becoming present in sufficient quantity to wipe out critical parts of the immune system, allowing horrible infections to take hold. The new treatments for HIV kill many but not all of the virus particles. But since the viral load gets smaller and smaller, immune function can return to normal and symptoms disappear. What is exciting about medical advances in this field is that research doctors pretty much understand how the antiviral medicines work, and so they can work to develop new and more potent medicines to kill HIV itself.

But AIDS is unusual in medicine because we know its cause—HIV. In contrast, other diseases rarely have a single cause. Take heart disease as an example. In the nineteenth century, doctors learned that atherosclerosis, or clogging of the arteries in the heart, was a common cause of heart attack and heart failure. The twentieth century brought the understanding that nutritional factors related to eating fatty foods increased the risk of a person's getting atherosclerosis and heart disease. But the twenty-first century has brought other factors into focus—for example, that a smoldering infection can occur within the walls of coronary vessels, and the resulting inflammation can lead to clogging of the vessel.

Even though the cause of coronary artery disease remains unclear, we can use medicines to treat the heart when it develops problems pumping blood due to heart failure. When that happens, the heart's inability to pump blood forward throughout the body leads to a backup of blood. This pooling of blood can lead to leg swelling and difficulty breathing—a condition known as congestive heart failure, or CHF. Doctors have recognized the clinical syndrome of CHF for many years, and they have had an armamentarium of drugs to deal with this syndrome. A great example is digitalis. The original source of this drug was a plant called foxglove. Doctors in the seventeenth century learned that foxglove tea would relieve the leg swelling and shortness of breath that a century later would be named congestive heart failure.

Another common example is aspirin. Take it when you have a fever, and your body temperature will start to drop, leaving you feeling better. So even if the exact cause of the problem is not known, medicines do exist to help relieve the discomfort caused by the symptoms and by the underlying illness.

## How Drugs Help Explain Unexplained Illnesses

The doctor's idea that patients who have symptoms without a medical explanation have "nothing wrong" with them changes when a medicine hits the market that removes the symptoms. Now the person can, in essence, be cured of an illness that—according to some doctors—didn't exist just a short time before. Irritable bowel syndrome (IBS), one of the conditions we've looked at in this book, is a great example. Two medicines have recently come onto the market for women with IBS. The first is alosetron (Lotronex) and is given to women whose IBS is "diarrhea predominant." The FDA took alosetron off the market after reports of severe gastrointestinal side effects, including gut perforation and even death. But the drug was so effective in relieving the diarrhea in women with diarrhea-prominent IBS that women lobbied successfully for its reinstatement, albeit under carefully monitored conditions to reduce side effects. The second is tegaserod (known by the brand name Zelnorm) and is given to women whose IBS is "constipation predominant," meaning that constipation is the main symptom they experience. Interestingly, the FDA just took tegaserod off the market because of an increased risk for heart attack or stroke. IBS support groups are already up in arms. Only time will tell if patient demands will somehow balance the newly discovered risks, allowing the drug to become available again, even if only limitedly.

Although the cause of IBS is not known, researchers do know that movement of food through the intestines is under the control of autonomic nerves to the gut, and serotonin is an important player in that control. I have discussed serotonin before as a substance related to depressed mood and to pain. In IBS, the normal tone of the gut serotonin system is turned up, sometimes by stress and sometimes by infection, causing abdominal pain and diarrhea. Tegaserod and alosetron have exactly opposite effects on the serotonin system: tegaserod tends to turn it on and relieve constipation, while alosetron tends to block it and relieve diarrhea.

Interestingly enough, if we test a person with IBS, in most cases we'll find nothing wrong; no abnormality in the gut muscle, no infection, and no chemical imbalance, for example. And yet here are two drugs that work to substantially relieve the patient's symptoms. Obviously *something* was wrong if drugs work to make the patient more comfortable. So finding two drugs that act in opposite directions on the serotonergic nervous system, and which greatly relieve the wide range of bowel-related IBS symptoms, supports the hypothesis that IBS is caused by dysfunction in the serotonin system—that is, "something wrong."

The development of drugs like these leads to the prediction that medicine is about to make a critical turn. It's reasonable to say that chronic fatigue syndrome (CFS), fibromyalgia (FM), and IBS are "functional illnesses" in that there is no evident pathology. But it's no longer okay to equate "functional" with "all in your head." The efficacy of these drugs in relieving the symptoms of these medically unexplained syndromes means that they are, in fact, real diseases.

## Primary Drug Treatments for Fatigue

Fatigue, and the brain fog that accompanies it, can be hard to treat because there are as yet only a few drug options. But some drugs do exist, including a few that you might not think of as drugs. For example, when I discussed narcolepsy earlier, I noted that caffeine is the simplest treatment available. But while caffeine can be useful in cases of mild fatigue, many people are very sensitive to other symptoms produced by this general stimulant—the feeling of nervousness, of their heart pounding, or the need to urinate over and over again. Another medicine that helps some patients feel better is vitamin $B_{12}$, given in large doses by injection. One study done many years ago did suggest that it could improve general well-being, but with only limited effects on fatigue. Medical students are taught that vitamins are useful only in patients who, for one reason or another, have a vitamin deficiency. However, enough patients have reported that vitamin $B_{12}$ is helpful that I am willing to try this, especially because this vitamin is not toxic and costs so little. Moreover, one study found evidence of lower than normal levels of this vitamin in the spinal fluid of patients with CFS.

To ensure vitamin absorption, I teach relatives or friends how to give the vitamin by injection, which is simple to do. Although the standard available dose of 1,000 units per milliliter is probably sufficient, Hopewell Pharmacy and Compounding Center (800-792-6670) makes a solution with a high concentration of 5,000 units per milliliter, and I instruct the patient to receive a 1-milliliter injection two to three times a week.

When I turn to prescription medicines for fatigue, the first I try is modafinil (Provigil). I described this drug in my discussion of sleep in the last chapter, because it is FDA-approved for the excessive sleepiness associated with chronic pathological conditions. These include narcolepsy, sleep apnea, and moderate to severe cases of a condition known as chronic shift work sleep disorder, which gets its name from the severe sleepiness some night shift workers feel. The advantage of modafinil over general pharmacological stimulants is that it targets the brain regions controlling sleep and wakefulness while not affecting those sites responsible for addiction. This enhanced specificity greatly lowers the risk of abuse. In contrast, more broadly active stimulants have a market on the street because they lack this specificity as is evident from effects that can include euphoria. When drugs produce emotional highs or lows, they are usually habit forming. Modafinil is not.

I helped conduct a double-blind, placebo-controlled trial of modafinil in CFS that involved five different medical centers. It's worth explaining what this means, since you're liable to see many references, in ads for prescription drugs and in medical journals, to drug trials of this kind. Sick people tend to feel better when receiving treatment of any kind. A century or more ago, medical researchers learned that giving patients even a sugar pill—one that looks identical to the drug being tested but has no real effect—could make some patients feel better. So in order to figure out how effective a new drug is in reducing symptoms, researchers compare its effect against that of a placebo: a sugar pill. Since every patient in a placebo-controlled trial gets some treatment, this type of study allows the researcher to sort out the therapeutic effect of the active drug, comparing its effect to that of just being treated with an inactive substance. A double-blind study is one in which neither the patient nor the prescribing doctor knows whether the "drug" being taken is, in fact, the real drug or the placebo. This double-blind design turns out to be critical to remove the slightest doubt that the researcher might telegraph information about the contents of the pill to the patient; obviously, if this were to happen, the integrity of the study would be in question, as would any positive results. For this design to work, a person should not have any cues as to whether he or she is on the drug or the placebo. Both have to look and taste alike and produce similar side effects. So if, for example, the actual drug tinged your vision yellow, and you talked with other participants in the drug trial who didn't have this side effect, you might quickly figure out that you were on the active drug. Whether or not it were true, your believing that you were on the active drug by itself could make you feel better and thus confuse the actual end result.

One unfortunate reality of drug trials is that the company sponsoring the research usually wants the results yesterday. After all, trials cost money, and pharmaceutical companies want a quick answer to the question: Does the drug work? The results of the modafinil trial show why using a placebo is so important.

In our study, a large number of patients were involved at two sites and a smaller number at three other sites, including our own. The sites that had tested the most patients had a huge placebo effect. In fact, CFS patients at those two sites felt better taking the sugar pill than they did taking the active drug! I'm not sure just what the doctors at those sites did and said to get this striking placebo response, but I would like to bottle it. In my experience and that of others, seeing striking improvement of fatigue with any drug is rare, let alone finding those results with a sugar pill.

The remaining sites—including our own—showed the opposite tendency, but the numbers of patients recruited were too small to outweigh the negative effect from the other two sites. I've told you this story to make the point that the gold standard for drug testing can have flaws that muddy the water. Although the negative results of this study could mean the drug is not helpful in treating fatigue, I think a follow-up study should be done that will address the shortcomings of the first one. I have used modafinil for several years now and am convinced that the drug has benefits, but only for some people. Proving that is an important goal, as is determining why some patients react differently from others.

About half the patients who use this drug tell me that it does not help their fatigue at all. Of the remaining half, half again have side effects—nervousness, headache, more fatigue—that make it problematic to continue taking the drug. The other quarter of patients *do* seem to benefit. The take-home message is that this particular treatment for fatigue is nothing like using penicillin to treat a strep throat. In that case, the results of a placebo-controlled, double-blind trial would be clear. The sore throat would quickly go away on active drug, while there would be relatively little effect from the placebo. Here the results are muddier.

For now I'm willing to try modafinil, at least for six weeks. I prescribe 200 mg tablets and have the patient start with half a pill. If the patient tells me he or she has problems with most drugs, I will prescribe the 100 mg tablets and have the patient start with half of one of those. If the patient feels a lot better after taking the drug, we maintain that dosage. If there is no effect, I may prescribe a second dose to be taken no later than 1 p.m. (taken later in the day, the drug might disturb sleep). In cases where we find an acceptable dosage that reduces fatigue, patients continue to take it and the effect usually continues over time.

When modafinil does not work or produces intolerable side effects, I will try a general stimulant such as methylphenidate (Ritalin). This is the same Ritalin that became well known in reducing hyperactivity in children. Methylphenidate may calm hyperactive children, but in some adults it helps combat fatigue. No one really understands why the drug has diametrically different actions in children and adults. This class of drugs is under strict control because of its abuse potential. However, this has not been an issue in my patient population.

A recent double-blind placebo-controlled trial did find this drug to reduce fatigue and improve concentration. I start with 5 mg once a day and then, if needed, add a second, lunchtime dose. If there are no side effects and no definite effect, I will gradually increase the dose to as high as 20 mg twice a day. At this point, I may move to one long-acting dose, but I rarely go beyond this dose.

An alternative to modafinil is an amphetamine. This class of drugs was used by the U.S. Army to offset fatigue before modafinil was developed. An early study showed that it could be useful in treating CFS. Despite this, amphetamines have a slew of side effects, starting with addiction and the other side effects we've already discussed, sometimes even producing agitation. However, some people who cannot tolerate Provigil or Ritalin do just fine on an amphetamine. With this drug, I use as little as is necessary to produce a noticeable reduction in the patient's fatigue.

To my amazement, some insurance companies insist that patients try methylphenidate or amphetamines before they will pay for modafinil, even though these drugs can have much more serious side effects. Modafinil is not yet on the list of drugs the FDA has approved for use in chronic fatigue syndrome or idiopathic chronic fatigue (ICF), although it's approved for other purposes. Not allowing a person to take this drug is clearly backward thinking, but insurers also don't cooperate because modafinil is more expensive than stimulants that have been on the market for many decades. Although reducing health costs is important, making people take potentially dangerous drugs simply because they're less expensive than the alternatives is a mistake.

In the past, and occasionally still today, I prescribed another drug that is usually used in the treatment of Parkinson's disease, an illness in which fatigue is often prominent. Selegeline (Eldepryl) also appears to have a role in the treatment of fatigue that is unrelated to Parkinson's. Selegeline is an MAO inhibitor, one of the class of drugs we discussed in chapter 5, but, at therapeutic doses of 5 mg twice a day, it doesn't have the toxic "cheese effect" I described there. Since it has no antidepressant action at all at these doses, it is not used in the treatment of depression. I decided to try it in CFS when I learned that the selegeline molecule resembled an amphetamine. My other reason for wanting to try an MAO inhibitor related to the overlap between CFS and atypical depression that I laid out in chapter 5. I did a trial of selegeline in a small number of CFS patients and found a very small but positive effect.

So for individuals who do not respond well to modafinil or the other stimulants, I would try selegeline. Importantly, however, there is a new transdermal version of selegeline (Emsam) that can be used to treat depression. Putting the drug into the body through the skin allows for higher blood levels without the risk of the cheese effect. I expect this version of selegeline to work better than the oral version I have used. The downside of using it is that it is expensive. Nonetheless, I plan to start using this drug in my practice while waiting for FDA approval of new oral MAO inhibitors that have antidepressant action without the cheese effect. These could be an important new avenue for treatment in that one report supports using such drugs in reducing fatigue in CFS.

One drug that was reported to reduce severe fatigue is hydrocortisone, an anti-inflammatory hormone made within the body. You've probably encountered hydrocortisone before, since it's used as a popular treatment for itchiness and other skin inflammations. For those purposes, it's sold in very low doses as a topical cream. When patients have autoimmune diseases, on the other hand, doctors often treat patients with very high doses of these steroids taken as pills. The report showing efficacy of hydrocortisone on fatigue was remarkable in that very small amounts of this drug—actually substantially less than the body itself makes—reduced symptoms in a double-blind placebo-controlled trial. Unfortunately, a follow-up trial was not effective. I have tried low-dose hydrocortisone therapy on about twenty patients with no remarkable success. On occasion, I will still try it, especially when patients also complain of muscle pain and/or if they have elevated antinuclear or anti-thyroid antibodies—signs of possible inflammatory or autoimmune disease. Such patients fall through the cracks of medicine because they do not fulfill diagnostic criteria for autoimmune disease, but on occasion such a patient does feel a lot better on steroids. This successful outcome means that the person probably does have an autoimmune disease causing the symptoms.

Back in the 1980s and 1990s, many doctors believed that disabling fatigue was likely due to a problem with the immune system (called *immune dysregulation*). Because of this, they sometimes prescribed intravenous gamma globulin in patients with severe cases. However, a well-done double-blind placebo-controlled trial showed this treatment to be ineffective. There are still two times, however, when this treatment is worth considering. Reductions in some of the body's immunoglobulins can produce a mild immune deficiency, associated with repeated episodes of infection like a sore throat, bronchitis, or pneumonia. If I have a patient with a history of repeated infection as well as reduction in several subclasses of immunoglobulin G, I will try intravenous gamma globulin. I would also consider using this treatment if an ongoing viral infection can be documented—very rare in my experience.

Another immune modulator that may help severe fatigue is a drug called Ampligen, which must be given intravenously and will probably be costly. FDA approval for this drug awaits the results of a recently completed large multicenter trial testing its efficacy in CFS. Preliminary results are not terribly promising, however. One very interesting trial reported that weekly injections of another immune stimulant improved the symptoms of pain and fatigue in patients with no medical explanation for their symptoms. Unfortunately, the immune stimulant was a vaccine that is not available in the United States.

## Drugs for Chronic Pain and the Natelson Six-Week Rule

Widespread bodily pain is the other major symptom that I deal with in my practice. It is such a common and often disabling symptom that pain management centers have sprung up all over the United States. But you may not have such a center in your own community, so here I want to lay out the protocol I use to help people deal with their chronic widespread pain. You should plan to share this protocol with your doctor.

*Step 1.*    Most doctors first try a class of medicines called *nonsteroidal anti-inflammatory drugs* (NSAIDs), many of which are available without a prescription. You're already very familiar with many of them—the most commonly used drug in this class is that tried-and-true favorite, aspirin. Next is ibuprofen (often known by brand names like Motrin or Advil). Carefully done trials of this class of drugs in fibromyalgia (FM) have not shown a clear therapeutic effect, but many of my patients swear by them. The major toxicity from this class of drugs is gastric upset.

A new class of NSAIDs called *Cox-2 inhibitors* was developed to reduce this side effect. However, a number of large studies have found that these newer drugs have a higher rate of potentially lethal side effects, such as heart attack or stroke, than the old fashioned NSAIDs. Two of them—Vioxx and Bextra—have been taken off the market. Although Celebrex is still available, I think its risk for people taking it chronically outweighs any potential benefit over ibuprofen. Whether these toxicities extend to the older class of NSAIDs is currently not known but is a question undergoing research.

When I recommend NSAIDs, I'm actually ignoring the fact that no good evidence exists for their use in reducing FM pain. However, in my experience, a substantial number of patients reporting muscle and joint pain indicate relief when using this class of drugs. So I try them as the first step in my pain management regimen, and I apply what I like to call the Natelson Six-Week Rule. If the patient cannot tell me the drug has *definitely* helped reduce pain at the end of a six-week trial period, I will discontinue its use. Six weeks is long enough to know whether a drug has had a beneficial effect, and it can be pointless—or in some cases even detrimental—to continue taking a drug unnecessarily. Many chronic pain sufferers first arrive in my office with a suitcase full of medicines, unclear on how long they've been taking them or whether to keep on using them. In that case, I start slowly removing medicines, one at a time. Sometimes, this "drug holiday" helps by itself; other times, stopping the medicines produces no effect except on the patient's pocketbook. One thing is certain: once you're on several medications, it's important to have a doctor's supervision when you start to discontinue them.

*Step 2.*   A brand-new drug promises to do for FM what Lotronex and Zelnorm did for IBS—that is, make doctors take FM seriously. I mentioned this drug—duloxetine or Cymbalta—in chapter 5 because it is an antidepressant. Its availability has changed the way

I manage pain; beyond the NSAIDs, it's usually the first one I try to relieve widespread pain, regardless of whether the patient is depressed.

Duloxetine is a twenty-first-century version of an older class of antidepressant drugs called tricyclics, but with substantially fewer side effects. Like the tricyclics, duloxetine interferes with the uptake of both serotonin and norepinephrine and is therefore known as a *serotonin/norepinephrine reuptake inhibitor* (SNRI). Duloxetine is the first in that class of drugs shown by double-blind placebo-controlled trials to have two separate and independent actions: pain relief and depression relief. Specifically, it has proven successful in relieving both widespread FM-type pain as well as the neuropathic, burning pain that occurs in feet and hands due to the effect of diabetes on peripheral nerves, and it does this whether or not depression is present. The pharmaceutical industry realizes that pain is a huge market, and the value of the drugs in this class in relieving FM pain has spurred other companies to work on developing new drugs. You, the consumer, will benefit from this change in attention. Moreover, the development of drugs specifically to relieve FM will at last revolutionize the way physicians think of the syndrome. As we saw with IBS, when treatments exist that really work, skeptics can no longer argue that the problem is "all in your head."

Another advantage to this class of drugs is that the same dose that relieves pain also relieves depression. Treating depression, when it is present, often has the additional effect of reducing pain. In fact, several carefully done placebo-controlled studies have shown that antidepressant treatment can improve some FM symptoms as well as improving quality of life. With SNRIs, the opposite is also true: treating the pain of FM can also help relieve depression. What is unclear in all these studies is the role of depression in worsening pain and fatigue, but using these drugs bypasses that question. When the depression lifts, you'll feel better and be more able to cope with your pain. That, of course, may also help *eliminate* the pain.

Prior to duloxetine's becoming available, my second step in treating pain was to use low doses (10 mg to 25 mg) of the old-fashioned tricyclic antidepressants (TCAs). This early class of antidepressants has similar dual actions on serotonin and norepinephrine and also relieves FM pain, but with significant side effects including a very dry mouth, a fast heart rate, constipation, and, all too often, weight gain in women. Despite these side effects, I still use these as my first line drug for pain in three kinds of cases: when money is an issue (duloxetine is very expensive, but TCAs are cheap); major problems with recurrent headaches, for which low doses of TCAs often work wonders; and when the patient reports both pain and disrupted sleep. Sedation is a side effect of one drug in this earlier class, amitryptilene—sometimes known by the brand name Elavil—and so it can help with sleep problems. The other drugs in this class— nortryptilene (Pamelor) and desipramine (Norpramin)—are less sedating but still very effective in headache. When Elavil is too sedating, I will try Pamelor. And I will turn to Norpramin if for some reason the person has problems with duloxetine.

Some doctors use a class of drugs called muscle relaxants instead of the tricyclics. Double-blind placebo-controlled trials have established that TCAs, as well as a muscle relaxant called cyclobenzaprine (Flexeril), help to reduce FM pain. Flexeril's chemical structure resembles that of Elavil, and it is also sedating, though with the same set of side effects. So if a patient is already taking Flexeril and reports that it is improving sleep and/or reducing pain, I do not switch to a drug like Elavil. Flexeril probably works because of its resemblance to Elavil, but it is marketed for relief of muscle spasms.

Physicians probably started using Flexeril for the same reason they referred FM patients to rheumatologists: because they believed that FM was a disease of muscle and ligaments. There is little evidence for that line of thinking today, but one fortunate by-product of this old idea was the discovery that Flexeril could help treat chronic pain. This drives home an important point: sometimes drugs have many actions besides the ones for which they are marketed. And that can be a double-edged sword. Take, for example, another well-known muscle relaxant, diazepam, which is even better known by the brand name Valium. Besides being a muscle relaxant, Valium is also a general relaxant in that it reduces anxiety and helps some people with insomnia to fall asleep. And yet I never prescribe Valium, because no one knows whether the drug remains effective as a sedative if taken for more than a few days. What *is* well known, however, is that people can get chemically dependent on drugs in this class. Instead, I sometimes turn to a different muscle relaxant, tizanidine (Zanaflex). This drug is known to have pain-reducing properties, and one study (done, unfortunately, without a placebo control) suggested that the drug reduced FM pain. I have tried it, and patients report that it helps reduce their pain. Because of this, I will often try this drug in addition to duloxetine or the TCAs, or I will use it if the patient cannot tolerate one of these other medications.

*Step 3.*    When the drugs already mentioned are not enough to make pain tolerable, the next step is to add the antiepileptics. Let me make it clear that I do not use this class of medicines because chronic pain has anything to do with epilepsy, but because these drugs really do help reduce pain. Also, several of them have succeeded in relieving FM symptoms in double-blind placebo-controlled trials. Moreover, my own experience with antiepileptics has been positive, and their side effects are fairly minimal. One nice side benefit is that they often reduce headaches, too.

The first one I use is gabapentin (Neurontin). It is inexpensive and helpful in reducing pain in some patients, although it's not the easiest drug to work with. It has a short half-life and must be taken four times a day, and—although it's not really very effective as a sedative, especially at small doses—it can induce sleepiness. A new and cleaner version of this drug, called pregabalin (Lyrica), has recently been FDA-approved for some forms of pain. A double-blind placebo-controlled trial has shown its effectiveness in FM, and it was approved in June 2007 for FM—the first such approval. I have made it a part of my pain management program if the patient's finances allow. Other advantages of this drug is that it appears to also relieve anxiety and is taken only twice a day, thus making taking it less of a burden for patients with brain fog.

If the patient is getting partial pain relief on Neurontin or Lyrica, I will add a second antiepileptic working on a different pain-relieving system. In the past, I used a drug called lamotrigine

(Lamictal). But because it has a rare risk of serious skin allergy, I usually first use a more benign drug such as oxycarbazepine (Trileptal). The advantage of both these drugs is that they need to be taken only twice a day. When the patient is overweight and requires pain management, I often try topiramate (Topamax) or zonisamide (Zonegran). These antiepileptics have more side effects than the other ones; one of these is slight nausea, which helps reduce food intake and thus can lead to weight loss. But sometimes other side effects, like more fatigue and brain fog, limit the usefulness of these drugs.

*Step 4.*   This step starts with a painkiller called tramadol (Ultram). When used on top of the antiepileptics, it can often reduce FM-induced pain to tolerable levels. If there is minimal pain relief or if the patient reports feeling too drugged, I stop these drugs and move on to long-acting opiates—either methadone, a drug called MS-Contin, or an opiate pain patch (Duragesic). While the majority of women with widespread pain don't require step 4, there is clearly a need for opiates for *some* patients with chronic pain. However, opiates are famously habit-forming for a reason, and I don't prescribe them without first establishing what I call a "therapeutic alliance" with my patient. We agree that only one doctor writes the prescription for this class of drugs—either me or the primary-care provider. That allows me to know exactly how the patient is doing at all times.

Most primary-care doctors don't know about the long-acting opiates and instead prescribe short-acting ones like oxycodone with acetaminophen (a combination drug known by the brand name Percocet). The increased addiction potential of this class of drugs if taken long-term is the reason I *never use them* in my chronic pain management regimen. If you are taking this drug, I urge you to ask your doctor about referring you to a physician expert in pain management or at least have him or her read this chapter.

### Other Drugs for Pain

On occasion, I try other medicines before moving to opiates. For people with substantial tenderness in the neck, shoulders, and back, I sometimes try injections of a drug similar to the one used by your dentist to numb up your teeth before fixing a cavity. This is a short-acting anesthetic agent that I mix with a longer-acting one and a drop of an anti-inflammatory steroid. I do this on a trial basis. Sometimes, a patient reports that this procedure lessens the pain for days to even weeks. Then I make these injections part of that patient's pain management regimen. Some people with more localized pain find relief from skin patches that release into the skin a drug like the injectable numbing medicine.

In my opinion, some FM and CFS patients have a rheumatological disease causing achy muscles or joints, but without the swollen or red joints that a rheumatologist would use to make a diagnosis. Lab test results can reveal an underlying rheumatological disease. Some of my patients have sedimentation rates well above the normal of 20 and antinuclear antibodies (ANAs) levels of 1:320 or higher, which is well above the normal of 1:40. These test results point to an underlying autoimmune disease process. But without swelling and redness and without confirmatory tests for systemic lupus erythematosis (SLE) or other collagen vascular diseases, the rheumatologist passes. He or she won't say there is "nothing wrong" but rather "I don't think this is rheumatological disease." The result, once again, is that the patient falls through the cracks of classical medicine.

In my view, cases like these at least suggest trying drugs that rheumatologists might prescribe. One reason that rheumatologists may be hesitant to make a diagnosis of rheumatological disease is because of the toxic side effects of the drugs they use. After all, every time a doctor prescribes, he or she balances the risk of using the drug with its potential benefit. I deal with this issue in two ways. First, I view my use of any of these drugs as a trial with the goal of definite improvement within a one-month period. Second, I use steroids, a class of drugs in use for decades with broad anti-inflammatory actions, rather than some of the newer, less broadly acting drugs. If the pain disappears during this therapeutic trial, we would have all the more evidence of an underlying autoimmune disorder, since there is no

evidence—either in the literature or in my own experience—
that these drugs improve primary FM. To me, improvement
on steroids means the FM is secondary to an underlying autoimmune disease. A positive therapeutic trial puts me on the phone
to my rheumatologist colleague so that we can get on the
same page.

A second potential line of treatment may seem unusual at first
but employs a drug that's best known for fighting malaria. In
World War II, soldiers in the Pacific were given the antimalarial
drug Atabrine to take daily. Three side effects were quickly
noticed: the soldiers' skin turned yellow; they reported fewer
aches and pains; and they reported having more energy and less
fatigue. Subsequent research indicated that the drug had anti-
inflammatory properties, leading to a role for it in managing pain-
related symptoms in diseases of the joints and muscles. Since
Atabrine had other serious toxicities, however, it is no longer
available.

But rheumatologists routinely use a related but less toxic drug
called Plaquenil. We don't know whether this antimalarial relieves
fatigue, but it does help reduce muscle and joint inflammation,
typically after several months of use. If my patient doesn't report
a substantial improvement after three months, I'll stop this drug.
Since it can have a detrimental effect on vision, I will also have an
ophthalmologist check the eyes before I start this medicine, and
recheck them every six months thereafter.

### Other FM Therapies

A number of initial reports point to other potential therapies for
widespread pain with multiple areas of tenderness. People whose
bodies produce a low level of growth hormone (GH) may experience low energy, poor cognition, and an impaired ability to exercise. Researchers studied what it would be like to administer
additional growth hormone to FM patients whose bodies secreted
only a low level of GH. The hormone did help reduce FM symptoms but with some problems: it was expensive, it had to be given
by injection several times a week, it took six months to produce a
noticeable effect, and—most important—the improvements sim-

ply weren't dramatic. FM patients still had FM. And a similar trial with CFS patients had no effect at all.

Another study stemmed from the report that a drug used to relieve nausea helped reduce fatigue in severe liver disease. A recent double-blind placebo-controlled trial indicated that a drug in this class, tropisetron, could relieve FM pain. Interestingly, this drug has the same mechanism of action as alosetron, the selective $5\text{-HT}_3$-receptor antagonist used in treating diarrhea-predominant IBS. So while tropisetron does not appear to be helpful for gastrointestinal pain, it may help widespread pain. If the drug company making this product can convince the FDA of its efficacy, it should become available for use by your doctor.

Finally, there are positive preliminary results from an immune active substance—low doses of interferon-alpha given under the tongue. While tenderness at specific points in the body did not change, FM patients who were on the active product reported improved physical function relative to those on placebo. High doses of injected interferon are currently part of the standard treatment for hepatitis C, but oral preparations are not currently FDA-approved. If and when they are, they may gain a role in treating the diffuse achiness reported by patients with CFS and FM.

## Drugs for Disrupted or Unrefreshing Sleep

This symptom is very disturbing. The person reports that he or she lies in bed all night but can barely sleep. Disrupted sleep is a treatable symptom, but unfortunately treating it rarely relieves symptoms of chronic fatigue or widespread pain, and patients still complain of feeling unrefreshed when they awaken. It's understandable that people are often terribly upset by sleep difficulties and ask for relief.

Here's a case where products found at the health-food store can have a beneficial effect, at least for some people. You can start with tryptophan or melatonin. You may be familiar with tryptophan, or at least its effects, since it's present in your Thanksgiving turkey. Its most widely remarked (if indirect) effect is to lull you and your guests to sleep after holiday dinner. Tryptophan—or the product your body converts it into, 5-hydroxytryptophan (5-HTP)—can be particularly useful because these substances are part of the biochemical chain producing serotonin, a substance in the brain responsible for normal sleep. Although I usually prescribe only one dose before bed to aid sleep, a controlled study reported that taking 5-HTP three times a day led to improved sleep and less pain in FM patients. The second product is melatonin, a hormone that is also related to serotonin. Here dosage is an issue, with a group from the Massachusetts Institute of Technology suggesting that less was better. The problem with taking any of these food supplements, however, is that there is no regulation as to the amount of product in a pill and how much of it, when ingested, actually gets into the bloodstream. So one reason these supplements might not work is that there is either too little or too much melatonin in a tablet. Because of this, a new drug that acts like melatonin looks interesting. The drug, ramelteon (Rozerem), is FDA-approved for insomnia. This government approval means that consumers can be sure that the amount of drug stated on the packet is actually in the pill and that it has proven to be useful by a double-blind placebo-controlled trial. However, when the over-the-counter drugs don't work, this is not my next step. In late 2006, this drug cost a bit less than four dollars per pill.

My next step is to turn to the sedating antidepressants amitripyline (Elavil) or doxepin (Sinequan), which I've already described in other sections of this chapter. At low doses these make poor antidepressants, but they do help with sleep and pain. When the patient still reports disrupted sleep, I will try a sedative, usually fast-acting drugs like zolpidem (Ambien), zaleplon (Sonata), or the newest, eszopiclone (Lunesta). Although the drug companies push their newest product, one does not work any better than the next. Ambien will soon be available as a generic and provides the best overall effect of drugs in this group, so I prescribe it most often. Since the remaining drugs in this class are quite expensive and can also be habit-forming, my next choice is Rozerem, the melatonin-like drug I mentioned earlier, because it is the only one of the sleep-inducing drugs that is not habit-forming. If these are ineffective, I will try drugs in the benzodiazepine or Valium class, such as temazepam (Restoril) or clonazepam (Klonopin). I don't like using these drugs because patients often find it hard to stop using them, or even to reduce the dose. In fact, just tapering off the dose can result in a major-league rebound of insomnia and nervousness. But some patients report that this kind of drug helps reduce daytime fatigue. Once again, while some of the reasons for these effects are unclear, I'm willing to try these drugs in some cases.

If a drug works in a certain illness, that positive effect can tell us something about the biological processes producing the illness. For example, the successful outcome of a study on pharmacological doses of 5-HTP, one of the building blocks (the scientific word for this is substrate) for serotonin, the brain-active substance involved in sleep and pain indicates that some FM patients have sleep disorders. Several recent studies show that disturbing sleep in healthy people can lead to increases in musculoskeletal achiness and/or decreases in their pain threshold. To me, this means that some patients have a problem with sleep that adds up over time to produce the syndrome of FM. Although the exact nature of this sleep problem remains an issue for research, a carefully done placebo-controlled trial of a drug called sodium oxalate (Xyrem) did show it to help FM. The drug improved sleep and diminished pain in patients with widespread pain and tenderness. I have begun using the drug for FM patients with major sleep problems, with mixed results. Sometimes it is really helpful, and other times it does nothing.

Xyrem, however, is heavily controlled for a very good reason: when it was freely available, some men unfortunately used this powerful sedative as a tool for date rape. The FDA wisely decided to control its use, and now it is only available at one pharmacy in the United States. The drug company that makes Xyrem is in the midst of a large study on its use in FM. We will have to await the outcome of that trial before most practitioners will consider its use, but I am guardedly optimistic.

In addition to the real possibility that FM may be due to disturbed sleep, I strongly believe that some patients with medically unexplained fatigue may have a sleep disorder. My line of thinking has recently been supported by the National Institutes of Health, which is funding my study examining sleep in CFS patients (this is not a drug trial). I will discuss this more in chapter 11. But, if you are interested in finding out about my research activities and those of my colleagues at the New Jersey Medical School, check out our Web site, www.umdnj.edu/fatigue.

The bottom line, of course, is to decide if my treatment has allowed the patient to sleep without all the awakenings experienced in the past. I ask if the patient feels slightly more refreshed in the morning. If he or she answers no, then I discuss stopping the treatments.

## Drug Development

The explosion in successful treatments for IBS points the way to potential treatments for the other illnesses discussed in this book. Prior to the development of the IBS drugs, treatment for IBS was marginal at best. But with the success of the recently available drugs, IBS becomes a focus for drug development. Fibromyalgia is a close second. New treatments for FM are now on the market, and clinical trials for more drugs are ongoing. Pain management has become a subspecialty in medicine and is recognized as an area needing further drug discovery by the pharmaceutical companies. And all of these treatments for pain will undoubtedly have a positive impact on face and jaw pain, too.

Treatments for fatigue and brain fog lag behind, but, as I have indicated, a pharmacopeia does exist. One major problem of taking medicines for any medical problem is that their use often comes with side effects that limit the duration of time they remain useful. I can think of several patients who got substantial relief of fatigue with modafinil but had to stop the drug when it began disturbing their sleep. Other patients reported good results from my pain management protocol, but decided to stop the medicines due to side effects. Subsequently, these same patients reported more problems with pain but fewer symptoms of brain fog and fatigue. Using drugs is a double-edged sword: they can be beneficial both in the short and the long term, but they can sometimes complicate cases, or render treatment results unclear. Whenever it's necessary, as a physician, I am prepared to remove my patients from drugs, slowly of course, so I can try to sort out the helpful and the hindering components of their use.

All of this should help you realize that drugs are not the whole answer, at least not today. So while it would be great for the doctor to have a pharmaceutical cure for your fatigue and pain, this outcome happens only rarely. Fortunately, drugs are just one set of tools in the arsenal. As we'll see in the next chapter, there are alternatives that also work. But "alternative" is really not the right word. The treatments I will go into next really complement drug therapy. And they come with an advantage: they convert you from your previous role of passive patient into being an active participant on the road to wellness.

# 8

# Step Four: The Integrative Mind-Body Approach

In many ways, all of the drug treatments I discussed in the last chapter are just crutches. They reduce symptoms to a greater or lesser degree, but they only rarely get a disabled person back to work. While drugs may and probably will be part of the process of getting you well, they are only one part of the path to wellness.

Wellness is a process, and not necessarily an easy one when you're feeling lousy; but the good news is that you really can take control of your body. Certain techniques from rehabilitation medicine act as a major supplement to drugs and other parts of your course of treatment. In this chapter, you'll discover how to conserve energy throughout the day, and even engage in what I call "energy building." The purpose of this part of the program is to help you take charge of managing your activity.

Here is an example of what not to do. Barbara Laurelton, one of my patients, was a forty-two-year-old midlevel executive with chronic fatigue syndrome (CFS). Fortunately for her, sometimes she experienced periods of up to several days when she felt a lot better than usual. Through medical treatment, I was able to make these episodes occur more frequently. During one of these times of relative wellness, Ms. Laurelton decided to do some spring cleaning. Unfortunately, though, she chose an especially energy-intensive activity, and beat her rugs. That short burst of high-intensity activity put Ms. Laurelton back in bed. In fact, she was so frustrated by her slide back into exhaustion that she lost faith in her own treatment. It was understandable for her to feel that way; having begun to hope that her periods of energy would continue and even grow more frequent, Ms. Laurelton was terribly disappointed when she landed back in bed so soon. That made her resistant to moving toward the next step in her recovery, which was *really* too bad.

Ms. Laurelton was a victim of what is often called the yo-yo effect, and my plan for wellness works hard to prevent it from occurring. I'll have a lot more to say about the yo-yo effect later in this chapter and will provide steps to help you avoid it. But for now, we should look at the key components that can help you smooth out these terrible swings from heightened to greatly reduced energy levels: energy conservation and energy building. The purpose of energy conservation is to budget the energy available to you throughout the day, and the purpose of energy building is to help you build a suit of body armor that will protect you from what happened to Ms. Laurelton.

## The Energy-In, Energy-Out System

The principle behind energy conservation is something that Dr. Lenny Jason, one of the country's leading CFS researchers, calls the envelope theory. The theory goes like this. Anyone—healthy or sick—has just so much energy available for use in any single day. The hardest thing someone with a new onset of severe fatigue has to do is to learn how to budget the energy he or she does have. This is where the envelope comes in.

View the envelope as holding all of the energy you have available in the course of a day. The best way to figure out how much energy you are expending each day is to count your steps with a device called a pedometer. This is biofeedback in action. Because it will pay to be accurate in doing this, I recommend you go with the Yamax 701 pedometer, which has undergone the most testing and standardization. It is available over the Internet. Set the pedometer to give you two measures: the number of steps you take and the number of feet you walk during your day. Wear it on a belt on your waist, just above the middle of a leg. Each day, record the number of steps and the distance, and reset the pedometer. Chart your daily activity for about a week. If you're not doing any unusual activity, you will find that your daily step count doesn't vary a whole lot. The average of that number is your "energy out."

The number of steps or feet you walk per day is clearly lower than it was when you were well. Sedentary healthy people walk anywhere from 1,000 to 3,000 steps per day. Severely ill patients will never hit anything close to 1,000. Don't be concerned that your step count is lower than these numbers. Knowing the amount of energy you expend in an average day is simply a starting point—information you need so you can track your further progress.

Being aware of how much energy you spend is only one part of the equation. Now let's look at the other side: the total amount of energy available to you. For simplicity's sake, you can use the same measure, and estimate the amount of your available energy as the total number of steps available to you in a day. I know you may be concerned about this process, since simply standing in place may take up much of your energy, and stress may also be a factor. But some quantification is a lot better than nothing, at least for getting started.

After you have done these steps, answer these questions: Is the amount of energy available to you equal to the amount of energy you are expending? Or, alternatively, do you think you have less or more energy than you are actually expending?

If, for example, you estimate that you ordinarily need to take 500 steps a day, but have only enough energy available to take 400 steps, you've got an imbalance—what I like to call an "in-out" problem. I use this shorthand to look at the energy available to you in an average day (energy "in") and the energy you expend in an average day (energy "out"). In this case, your "in-out" problem is that you have energy for 100 fewer steps than you need to take.

If at the end of each day you are feeling totally wiped out, you probably do have this sort of imbalance, and you will probably have to reduce your energy expenditure so that it fits within your own energy envelope. But if you are not totally wiped out at the end of the day, this may mean that you actually have more energy in your energy envelope than you are expending. A reasonable thing to do is to adjust your activities to match your energy-out measures.

Don't worry, the point of this exercise isn't to lower your expectations. Instead, it's about getting your arms around your energy and activity levels, becoming familiar with them in a way you probably haven't had to do before, and using these simple estimates to gauge your progress as you begin to bring the energy-in and energy-out into sync. *Then* you can move on to getting well. This is a whole different strategy from the past. Back then you worried about how you felt. Now you're using the feedback from your own activity to gauge your body—its limits and abilities—to get well.

As you start monitoring your energy expenditure, you may see a pattern developing, and it may have to do with a specific activity, or even a specific person with whom you usually do that activity. Let's look at an example. One of my patients, Ellen Collens, is a disabled nurse practitioner who has only about 1,000 steps of energy available to her each day. Last Memorial Day, she agreed to walk around town with her niece to serve as the photographer for her Girl Scout troop. Ms. Collens prepared for this activity by doing a little energy budgeting. She cancelled all of her usual daily activities so she'd have enough energy for her walk. But by the end of the day, her pedometer revealed that my patient and her niece had walked over 5,000 steps—a distance of over two miles—over a three-hour period. This is a very good example of what I call an in-out disconnect. Yes, when she had to do it, she was able to put forth the effort, but the story here is the same as when Ms. Laurelton beat her rugs. Greatly exceeding the energy envelope, even if you can, creates problems. Ms. Collens was so exhausted that she experienced a bad case of the yo-yo effect, which sent her to bed for the rest of the weekend. Nonetheless, she told me she would never forget that Memorial Day.

The issue here is expending energy in a situation where you cannot control it. When you do activities alone, it is up to you to decide whether to continue or to stop, but when you're in social situations, sometimes the decision is not fully up to you. Should you cancel all of your social engagements in order to avoid an overexpenditure of energy?

No, this is not a good idea. Being on the wellness path requires you to maintain social ties and not be isolated, and so a better solution is to arrange social activities so they're not a *surprise*. If you know how much energy you're likely to expend in a given situation, you can budget the energy you have available. What's most important is that you be the one to control your energy expenditure, and not someone else. Being aware of the issue will help. Ms. Collens learned from her own experience and has told me she is now trying to get a better assessment of the energy requirement involved in social events before saying yes.

Spend several weeks fine-tuning your energy envelope. Get to the point where the energy available to you comes pretty close to matching your total energy expenditure in steps. Some days you may feel somewhat more energetic than others. In other words, the energy available in your energy envelope may vary from day to day, but not too greatly. After you are pretty comfortable with this process, start thinking about making adjustments to the energy expenditure side of the equation. If you're consistently expending more energy than you estimate you have available—and are feeling the effects—you'll have to cut back. Charting your energy expenditure may allow you to notice if some particular activity uses up a lot of your available energy in a relatively small amount of time. Obviously you will have to compensate for this by expending less energy during the rest of that day. Being comfortable with your personal energy envelope will allow you to make these occasional adjustments.

What if the unexpected happens to you, as it did to Ms. Collens? Perhaps what you intended to be a brief trip to the market will turn into a several-hour affair. Just taking your kids to the park might cause you to expend more energy than you'd foreseen. You might have planned to sit on a bench watching your children in the playground, but you actually ended up playing with them or helping them interact with other kids. Similarly, recreational activities with your own friends are great but can lead to your being caught in a social situation where you're under pressure to continue when you really ought to stop. Simply being aware that you're embarking on an activity where the exact energy expenditure is unknown may allow you to budget better for the rest of your daily activities, and to back off if necessary. Both of these put you in control.

Remember Ms. Laurelton? Hers was an extreme example of overload, one she brought about all by herself. And it produced the "yo-yo effect plus." Her exertions put her to bed, and then she became afraid to try new activities. It took several appointments with me, consisting of nothing more than discussing this experience, until she got up the confidence to try my wellness regimen again. Ms. Laurelton's story is an accurate reflection of Lenny Jason's statement that "the yo-yo effect is a killer for people who have little energy. The key to helping the body to begin healing itself is to not put it on overload." Ms. Laurelton had put herself on overload.

The kind of activity that triggers this yo-yo effect varies with your state of wellness. If your total available energy is 700 steps, then spending an hour shopping for food, which involves driving, pushing a cart, and carrying many bags, could add up to over 500 steps, leaving you with little energy reserves for the rest of the day. So some patients with low energy reserves tell me on shopping days, the only other activities they do relate to personal hygiene. The point here is this energy yo-yoing over a very short period of time may exhaust your energy envelope and leave you little room for much else. And if you keep on going, this might make you sick.

If a healthy sedentary person takes a day off to go skiing, her energy expenditure will exceed the envelope of her available energy. The consequences of this won't be severe, but she'll be forced to change her usual behavior: she won't be able to go out that night but instead will have to go to bed early, and she may have to cut down on her activity the next day. Everyone—even someone who is perfectly well—can exceed his or her energy envelope at least on occasion. The consequences are different, though, for people with medically unexplained fatigue and pain. They're much more sensitive to the effects. So your primary goal on the first part of the road to wellness is to stay in your envelope. Know the amount of energy you have available, estimate (as best you can) the amount you're likely to need to spend, and try to avoid surprise expenditures.

Expect some "in-out" discrepancies until you get the hang of it. But you will succeed, and this will reduce symptom flare-ups and give you other pluses: improved sleep, a greater sense of control, and more energy over the long term. You should begin to see these effects within six weeks, and some people may see them substantially faster. When you achieve this goal, we can talk about increasing, or tipping up the end of, your energy envelope via a walking program that starts with a low energy expenditure and slowly raises your energy level.

If you've evaluated your energy envelope and find that you have more than 1,000 steps of energy available to you, you might be able to gauge your in and out energy levels all by yourself. But it's easier if you use the buddy system. Having a buddy who acts as a coaching partner to help you can make this process easier, shore up your resolve, and help you feel more secure in monitoring yourself. Remember, the lower the total amount of energy in your envelope, the greater the risk of the yo-yo effect. Ms. Laurelton was well on the road to recovery when she had her major crash. Since she went through this setback all alone, she became so frightened that she left the road to recovery altogether for a time.

A coaching partner can help you evaluate your energy expenditures so they match the energy available to you. Choose someone with whom you are close—a spouse or partner, a relative who lives nearby, or a close friend—and use him or her as a sounding board. Discuss your daily energy expenditures with this person and try to determine if they are reasonable, too high, or too low. If you and your partner think you can actually burn more energy, give it a try.

Review with your coaching partner the *way* you burn your energy. This only takes a few minutes, so don't worry about time. Do you burn a big portion of your available energy in one big burst? Or do you budget your energy to serve you throughout the day? You and your buddy should quickly see that expending a lot of energy in a small amount of time can lead to the yo-yo effect. Your coaching partner should help you distribute your energy expenditure more evenly throughout the day. The buddy system approach to managing energy within the envelope pays off. CFS patients who use the buddy system feel stronger and have more energy down the pike.

## Conditioning for Wellness

When you're facing constant fatigue, you learn to associate effort—any effort at all—with exhaustion. This associative learning is extremely strong. I have mentioned this before, and you may have heard this referred to as *Pavlovian conditioning*. Ivan Pavlov was a Nobel Prize–winning Russian biologist who lived from 1849 to 1936. His classic experiment showed that a dog could learn an association between an innocuous signal—the ringing of a bell, for example—and the availability of food. Eventually, just hearing a bell ring made Pavlov's dog salivate (a situation that's probably familiar to you if you live with a dog).

People really aren't very different from dogs in some ways, and this is one of them. Many of my patients with severe medically unexplained fatigue or pain report that just going through one or two pairings between exercise and illness flare-ups are enough to make them feel that any exercise at all would cause a worsening of their symptoms. Are they wrong? Not at all. Their symptoms are very real, and certain kinds of activity may, indeed, have made them even worse for a time. But what varies from patient to patient is what each does next. Some say to themselves, "I am going to cut way back on *all* my physical activity," while others say, "I am not going to do the type of activity that made me sick."

These are two very different responses. In the first, the person has become so frightened by the effects of exertion that he or she has decided to do much, much less. In the second example, the person realizes that certain activities carry a risk, but others may continue to be perfectly fine. Although the statements themselves don't sound all that different, they lay out dramatically different ways of looking at the relationship between activity and pain or fatigue. Moreover, they have everything to do with who each patient may be and where he or she is in life. But there is even more to the importance of personal characteristics. Some researchers believe that an individual's personal characteristics, habits, and beliefs influence whether a problem with pain or fatigue will follow an attack of a serious infection and become a long-term condition.

For example, studies have shown that individuals who have a tendency toward anxiety or depression or who tend to have a negative point of view about life are more likely to develop irritable bowel syndrome (IBS) after a bout of gastroenteritis. Similarly, the presence of fatigue or psychological distress just when some patients are also coming down with a sore throat and a cold predicts slowness of recovery and prolonged postinfectious fatigue. Furthermore, focusing on symptoms while believing that you can do nothing about them leads to delays in recovery.

We're not talking about microbiological studies that show how a germ can cause disease in a single person. Studies like the ones I've just cited instead describe tendencies over large numbers of people. This means that "person factors" are more important in influencing how some individuals feel and less important in influencing how others feel. Your friend might simply shake off increased achiness and fatigue after exertion, while your next-door neighbor might become quite concerned about the very same symptoms and decide to take a day off from work to rest. The point, however, is that deciding to engage in less activity can actually end up producing *more* symptoms, triggering a sort of vicious cycle. Deciding not to take that walk, because you remember how a shopping trip several weeks ago made you feel awful for three days, might actually make you feel less optimistic and less well. Budgeting your energy carefully and planning to take that walk tomorrow, however, might buoy your spirits and make you feel better—and never mind what happened several weeks ago.

Oddly enough, astronauts—some of the fittest people in the world—are completely familiar with this dynamic. When they return to Earth after being in space at zero gravity for as little as a week's time, astronauts nearly always become profoundly deconditioned. *Deconditioned* means that their bodies have suddenly become drastically out of shape. When these recently returned astronauts walk, they rapidly become exhausted. When they stand up, their normal cardiovascular reflexes work poorly, and they feel lightheaded and even faint. All this happens because astronauts in space live in an environment lacking gravity.

When researchers want to simulate living in a weightless environment while still on Earth, they don't exercise their volunteer patients to exhaustion: they put them to bed. After days of bedrest, these volunteers show the same kinds of biological changes as the astronauts. When they make even minimal effort, they feel their hearts pound and are very easily fatigued. Sound familiar? Prolonged resting may feel like the right thing to do; in fact, it may sometimes feel like the *only* thing you can do. But prolonged resting can also have adverse health effects well beyond producing more uncomfortable symptoms.

When I was an intern, the standard of care for someone with a heart attack was three weeks of bedrest. This prescription had two negative effects: it actually increased the rate of subsequent heart problems, and it made the heart attack survivor afraid of activity. Of course, nowadays we know that a carefully monitored program of aerobic activity protects against heart attacks.

If you're sick with fatigue and pain, your situation is surprisingly similar. If you decide to put yourself on bedrest, you'll be hit with a double whammy. Your illness, and maybe your learned response to previous activity, will make you less active. And then your need to rest will end up making you even more sick.

You're the one who can break this vicious cycle—not your doctor, not your use of drugs. You can use gentle physical conditioning to combat the biological changes that bedrest brings about. We now know that regardless of the disease, gentle physical conditioning reduces symptoms and improves quality of life. For elderly people who have trouble walking, for people awaiting cardiac transplant due to heart failure, for patients with multiple sclerosis (MS) or with medically unexplained pain or fatigue, a physical conditioning regimen helps rather than hurts—as long as it is done right.

When we know we have to do something, but we're afraid to do it, we can often find ourselves stuck. Fortunately, we can use a process called *cognitive behavioral therapy* (CBT) as an "unsticker." CBT was originally designed to be a treatment for depression and anxiety, but over time CBT practitioners have expanded the scope of their work. They learned they can work with people to improve how they cope with symptoms from any chronic illness, in effect to help them feel better. CBT, like gentle physical conditioning, is a treatment that reduces symptoms and increases the quality of life for people with a host of illnesses, including prominent severe fatigue and pain. Furthermore, CBT professionals can concentrate on specific symptoms like disturbed sleep with very good results. And if depression or stress is in the wings, the CBT professional can take care of those problems too, as we've already seen.

You can view CBT professionals either as therapists or wellness coaches. Finding such a coach and using CBT can be a critical step for anyone with medically unexplained illness. The CBT coach is an important part of my wellness team. CBT experts have the most experience dealing with stress, depression, and anxiety and relatively less experience in dealing with chronic medical illness. Even so, CBT is effective in reducing symptoms in half the patients who try it. So although absolutely everyone won't be helped by this therapy, at least 50 percent of people who spend eight to twelve sessions with an experienced cognitive behavioral therapist will feel substantially better. That kind of result makes trying CBT a must. And keep in mind that improvements you make while using CBT are in addition to those based on the medical approach I outlined in the last chapter. CBT is another step toward wellness.

What a shame medical schools don't have time to teach this kind of treatment. In fact, if I could change one thing in the modern medical school curriculum today, it would be to add a course on the principles of wellness therapy so it could be a part of every doctor's own personal therapeutic tool kit. Wellness therapy uses the strength of the doctor-patient relationship to help people with chronic illness feel better.

Here the key word is "better." If you were in my office, you would hear me say, "I can definitely help you, but I cannot predict whether you will be just a tiny bit better, somewhat better, or a whole lot better." Which of these will be the result depends on your own personal commitment to wellness and your willingness to trust the ideas behind wellness therapy. So really, even if I could fix the medical school curriculum, doctors wouldn't be the only ones who'd need to adopt this way of thinking. You, as a patient, have to buy into wellness therapy, too. We each have an important part to play. Together, you and your doctor can join forces to use everything that medicine and psychology have to offer to get you feeling better.

What factors, besides a fear of activity, can interfere with wellness? One is focusing too much on how you feel. Monitoring your symptoms and your feelings is normal, especially when you're sick. But there is a downside, especially if you spend a lot of time on this form of introspection. Focusing on how you feel every minute of every day, to the exclusion of other, more positive thoughts that are equally valid, often makes you feel worse.

If you need help freeing your mind to think of other things, try this. Make a list of pleasurable thoughts and activities you can still enjoy and that may be distracting in a good way. The next time you find yourself running a mental inventory of all your symptoms—for no other reason than habit—take out your list and choose something else to think about or do. Okay, you don't feel well; yes, you have a problem with achiness or fatigue. But you have positives in your life too, right? A grandchild, a video of a movie you love, a card game with friends. Work on developing your own list. All of these simple, pleasurable thoughts and activities can free your mind from a constant focus on your symptoms.

Here's the ultimate example. I'll never forget a forty-three-year-old patient, Doris Ellings, who arrived in my office with the surprising and happy news that she was pregnant. The baby changed her whole attitude about herself and her illness. Although Mrs. Ellings wasn't well, her symptoms diminished in intensity. Granted, nothing could be more distracting than a baby, and not every patient with chronic pain or fatigue will find herself prepared for pregnancy and childbirth. But the good news is that far less intense activities, and even training your mind to think pleasant thoughts, really can free you from the shackles of thinking *only* about your symptoms. The bottom line is to "accentuate the positive and eliminate the negative." Think of a few of your favorite things!

Illness is disempowering. Feeling sick without an obvious reason or an easy cure can make it seem that there is nothing you can do to help yourself. This sense of helplessness can interfere with wellness. But you can turn this around. Getting on the path to wellness is empowering. Making your available energy fit within your own energy envelope starts you on the path by putting an end to the yo-yo effect. The next step is to tip up the end of the energy envelope over time, gently increasing your daily activity. And this really works even for those people who feel they can do little beyond what they absolutely must to get through the day. When someone comes to my office and tells me he or she is walking regularly, I don't change the regimen but simply help manage and expand the current ones. Every patient in my practice who has conscientiously tried my regimen (or his or her own with my input) has felt better. That's 100 percent!

## Walking toward Wellness

To tip up the end of your energy envelope, you first have to save a bit of energy for some structured activity. The easiest is a bit of walking. Let's assume for a moment that you experience severe fatigue, but you've learned to balance your energy envelope at 800 steps per day—somewhat less than a quite sedentary but otherwise healthy person. Chose a small number of steps for a brief walk that you are pretty confident won't be a problem. Now plan to cut back on your energy expenditure by about 100 steps each day. Spend those saved steps on getting up and walking out of the house to the driveway. The goal is to keep the initial amount of activity small, so that it fits within your energy envelope. This puts you in control of your energy expenditure and prevents the yo-yo effect. It makes sense to bounce your choice off your coaching partner. Just plan to err on the conservative side. Here are some different scenarios for getting started with your walks, depending on your initial energy level.

## A Plan for Those with Low Energy Capacity

Especially if your energy envelope contains relatively few steps at first—fewer than 1,000, for example—you may initially feel winded, short of breath, or even more fatigued. Don't be frightened of these symptoms; they reflect your body's response to inactivity—the same thing those astronauts experienced. By exerting yourself just a little bit more than usual, any symptoms of added fatigue that do develop will not last long.

Then, instead of just walking to the start of the driveway, walk to the middle of the driveway (if you don't have a driveway, you could start by measuring a point several feet down your hallway or sidewalk). Yes, you might feel tired, but you'll bounce back as long as you've made room for this energy expenditure in your energy envelope. The gentle nature of this incremental activity will allow you to accomplish this slightly longer walk. You may need to stay at the same level for several weeks, but keep at it until it becomes a part of you. The next target will be the end of the driveway (or a point further down the hallway or sidewalk). Force yourself to be patient, adding activity in small increments. Fatigue has been a problem for a long time, and there is no reason to rush the recovery process. As you get comfortable doing this walking and more confident of your ability, add a second walk the same day, and later a third. Give yourself a *minimum* of ten days between increments.

So where do you go from here? If you were very inactive (pedometer readings of less than 700 steps per day), you should now be walking to the end of your driveway and back, two to three times a day. Walking slowly to the end of the driveway and back can take several minutes. Therefore, your total activity time will add up to be around 5 or even 6 minutes. Extend your distance 25 feet further; that should add another 10 to 15 seconds to your activity time. Be sure that you can fit this level of activity into your energy envelope. In order to do so, you may need to cut back on other activities to save some steps, at least initially. You will find that the total energy available to you in your energy envelope will slowly increase as you do more. This is a critical point to the wellness path. If you had to curtail one of your other activities in order to take your daily walks, you'll soon find you have enough energy to accomplish both.

Give yourself at least 10 days to incorporate this activity into your energy envelope. Then increase your distance by another 25 feet. Continue doing this slow incremental increase in walking distance until you get to three minutes of continuous activity. At that point, drop back to doing only two sessions per day. Continue to *slowly* increment your daily activity until you get to 5 minutes at a time; at this point, drop back to only one session per day. At this point, daily walking is no longer necessary. Move to an every-other-day (or a three-times-a-week) plan.

## Expanding the Energy Envelope

When you reach this point, reevaluate your daily activity. You'll be amazed that your energy envelope has expanded. Whereas you may only have been walking 500 steps on an average day, you'll be surprised to see that it is now more than that—maybe by only 10 or 20 steps but *more* nonetheless. This is what I mean by tipping up the edge of the energy envelope. This whole incremental process is step one in building a suit of "fitness armor" around yourself. When you're encased in this armor, you will be more resilient and will be able to do things that you have not done in months or even years.

Over the course of the next few months, you will slowly and gradually increase the amount of time you spend walking. By following this plan, you'll be filling the envelope with added energy— energy you can start to expend accordingly. By adopting a very gradual program of structured activity and keeping at it over time, your health and quality of life will slowly improve, and you will find yourself able to slowly increase your level of activity even further.

*Slowly* is the key word. Every person is different. You may have to wait for more than ten days before you lengthen your walk, or even feel you must stick at any one stage for up to a few weeks. But the critical thing is that you're taking control of your illness and fitting this additional activity into your own personal energy envelope. The envelope will prevent you from doing too much in any one session while strengthening your resistance to the yo-yo effect.

### For Those Starting with Higher Energy Capacity

Let's say you're starting from a slightly higher energy level—over 1,000 steps per day—or you've slowly increased the size of your energy envelope so that you've now arrived at this higher level. You can start with this same walking regimen until you're comfortable with the added activity. But you may be able to increase the length of your walks somewhat more quickly than if you started out with lower energy levels.

If your energy out value is 1,000 steps or more per day, start with the 5-minute program, three times a week, even if you suspect you could do more. Starting on the low side gives you a chance to integrate that activity into your energy envelope. Every step, even if small, puts you more and more in control and gives you confidence to move ahead with the program. If you have been sick for months to years, getting started is the important thing, not starting at a higher level.

Once you've reached this point, you'll be able to decide whether walking is for you or whether you want to choose a different activity. Walking is a relatively low-impact exercise that most of us can do around our own homes, without need of any fancy equipment. But some of my patients note that walking bothers their joints or backs. As an alternative, I often recommend they join an aquatics class, one especially designed for people with medical problems like rheumatoid arthritis. When you're in water, you weigh substantially less than you do on dry ground. Walking in a swimming pool actually relieves pressure on your back and reduces the strain of your foot hitting the ground. Some of my patients prefer to try to tread water or even to swim. This gentle version of aqua-fitness has been shown to help patients with fibromyalgia (FM). Remember while getting started that it's important to keep your level of activity to a minimum, giving yourself time to incorporate the new activity into your energy envelope. Once you find your ideal starting point, stick with that amount of activity until it is totally integrated into your energy envelope. Then you can begin ramping up, but slowly.

But let's return to the walking example. Now's the time to actively use your pedometer. Up to this point, you have used it to give you the total number of steps available in your energy envelope each day. Now, I want you to use it to give you the number of steps you take in your walk. Repeat this over a week or two. Your walk-related step count should remain about the same from day to day. Now increase your walking time by 15 seconds every 10 days. So instead of walking for 5 minutes, you will walk for 5 minutes and 15 seconds. Slow is good. If you have been sick for years, your progress is the important thing, not your speed. Ten days later, increase the length of your walk by another 15 seconds of duration. It will take you more than a month to get up to 6 minutes of walking. If you're starting with an energy level above 1,000 steps per day, you may be able to increase by 30-second increments every 10 days (or even every week), but it's always safer to try 15 seconds first, just to be sure that it will fit in your energy envelope.

As the duration of your walks increases, you will become more aware that your energy envelope is expanding. Make note of these changes, and continue this gradual incrementing process every week to 10 days. The next major milestone is 20 minutes. For some, getting here will take months, while others will attain this milestone faster. Either way, soon you'll be walking for a longer time, and taking more steps.

But—and this is important—even when you increase the length of your walks, you should still be walking slowly and no more often than three times a week. Twenty minutes is the magic number for reconditioning—the process needed to tone your muscles and your cardiovascular system. But in order to guarantee that this physiological process happens, you have to exceed 20 minutes. So gradually increase your walking duration to 30 minutes, still walking slowly, still walking only three times a week.

When you're comfortable walking for 30 minutes three times a week, you are firmly on the wellness path. Check out your energy envelope. Has your total step count increased again? If you are still making your walks three times a week, plus accomplishing all the other tasks you did when the walking program began, then the answer has to be yes. This means you have expanded your personal energy envelope. And you may even note that you have the energy available to accomplish a few other activities during the day, too. So success to this point puts you in control and adds positivity to your personal equation. Walking to wellness is a method that switches focus from the negative to the positive. It works for my patients and will work for you.

### For Those Starting with Normal Energy Capacity

Don't be put off by this subheading. While you may still have an energy problem, you have made short walks part of your weekly regimen. But this is also the entry point for people who don't have a major problem with severe fatigue. Take, for example, Connie Lowell, a thirty-seven-year-old veterinarian who came to see me about a five-year problem with achiness all over her body. On examination, she had fifteen of the eighteen tender points I reviewed with you in chapter 3. I diagnosed fibromyalgia. Despite her pain, she was able to live a relatively normal life. Dr. Lowell was less active than she had been prior to the onset of her pain problem, more tired at night, and less willing to do social activities than before. But still she considered her activity levels pretty normal for her.

Though her main complaint was pain and not fatigue, my walking regimen will still help Dr. Lowell. People with FM alone report that this walking technique considerably reduced their soreness. So if you are like Dr. Lowell, start a program of gentle walking lasting 30 minutes. Buy a pedometer to learn how many steps you walk in 30 minutes. Get in the habit of taking these walks three times a week. You may prefer to do these walks alone, but it might be more pleasant if you walked with a companion. Once you've made this part of your weekly routine, you are ready to take up the pace.

## Picking up the Pace to Wellness

Whether your difficulty is with pain, low energy, or both, you can now consider increasing the speed at which you walk. The 30-minute duration of your walks opens the door to biological toning, which is only just beginning when you walk at lower speeds.

This toning process directly combats fatigue and pain, so maximizing it is important. Your pedometer is a tool that can help you increase your walking speed, by giving you feedback on how many steps you're taking in your walks (your total step count) as well as the distance in feet that you've traveled. Increase your total step count by 25 steps and walk this distance in the same 30-minute duration that you have been doing. As was the case with the duration of the walk, take your time in increasing walking speed. A week to 10 days later, increase your speed by another 25 steps. Be sure you can fit the slightly increased energy expenditure into your energy envelope. You should be very comfortable in doing these assessments by this point. If you are not sure, just go slower. If you have a coaching partner, work with him or her so you can be clear about your energy envelope.

You will already have noted that your body provides you a rhythm for walking. As your right foot hits the ground, your left hand is in front of you. As your left foot hits, your right hand leads. Left foot, right hand; right foot, left hand. You will find yourself falling into a rhythm.

Now I want you to add words to the rhythm. These words are my "wellness mantra": "I'm better today than yesterday." As you pick up speed, you may find yourself streamlining these words so they sound more like: "M'better t'day than yestaday." If you prefer a different phrase, go ahead and use it; I want you to find a phrase that works for you and is positive. As a matter of fact, I urge my patients to say this to themselves the moment they open their eyes in the morning. Try it. It will start your day out more positively than without it. Saying these words when you awaken and during your walks is important because they are positives. Remember that positive thinking is part of getting well, while negative thinking just restarts that old vicious cycle again and makes you focus on your symptoms. Being positive leads to wellness.

The well-known writer Norman Cousins was sick with a severe rheumatological illness and used humor as a wellness tool. He discovered that maintaining a positive attitude, partly by using a massive helping of humor, made him feel better both physically and emotionally. Reciting your wellness mantra as you walk will make it easier for you to pick up your walking pace, and this will make you better. It's another kind of cycle, just not a vicious one.

Continue this gradual incrementing process by adding 25 steps every week to 10 days. Remember to keep your walking time to 30 minutes. Obviously it will take some practice to learn how to do this, but your pedometer will help. The next milestone is walking at 1 mile per hour—that is, half a mile in 30 minutes. Depending on your step length, that is about 1,000 steps. Remember back to when you totaled less than this in a whole day? This is progress!

Once you reach this milestone, you can increase your increments by 50 steps every week or 10 days. When you get to 2 miles per hour, you will still be walking at a comfortable pace. Now you can increase your increments by 100 steps every week or 10 days.

Susan Dobbs, a patient of mine, was able to follow the basic outline I have set out for the wellness path, until she hit 2.4 miles per hour. Every time she increased the speed on her treadmill to allow her to walk at 2.5 miles per hour, she developed achiness. At 2.4 she was fine; 2.5 seemed to be too much. So she came up with a novel solution: She walked at a speed of 2.5 miles per hour for just 1 minute and then set the speed back to 2.4 miles per hour for the remaining 29 minutes. On her next walk, she increased the 2.5 mile per hour duration to 2 of the 30 minutes. Slowly but inexorably, she got around what had seemed to be an impossible block. The take-home message from Ms. Dobbs's story is that you don't have to make a *complete* jump every time you go up on duration or speed. Her solution prevented the yo-yo effect and worked for her. After attaining 2.5 miles per hour for the entire 30 minute walk, she was able to continue to the final target speed—a brisk walk of between 3.2 and 3.5 miles per hour. Chose 3.5 if you are tall or are already feeling fine when you walk at 3.2.

When you use the program to get all the way to the speed of 3.2 miles per hour, your pedometer will show that you have walked 1.6 miles in the course of your 30-minute walk. That's over 3,000 steps for this single walk. Walking at this speed for 30 minutes will increase your heart rate and may make you sweat. Finding these signs of biological activation is good in that their presence leads to improved function and the ability to withstand small energy expenditures that used to produce the yo-yo effect.

Prove to yourself that your body is responding by taking your heart rate at rest and at the end of your walk. The simplest way to count your heart rate is by putting your index and middle fingers together under the crook of your neck, about an inch from the middle of your wind pipe. Count your pulse for 15 seconds and then multiply by four; for a slightly more accurate record, count for 30 seconds and multiply by two. Your resting heart rate may vary from 60 to 90 beats per minute. At the end of your walk, your heart rate should be at least 30 beats per minute faster than your heart rate at rest. Don't be frightened if your heart rate is higher; this is totally normal and simply reflects your own biological response to the toning stimulus.

Experiencing these physiological changes related to your walks indicates that your body is becoming more fit and is evidence that you're building the armor needed to allow you a better quality of life. Getting to this point will take many weeks and months, but if you create a diary of what you are doing every time you walk, you will see your progress. All you need to do is write down the date, how long you walked, and for what distance (or for how many steps). You will be impressed!

But what will most impress you is the fact that you now have an energy reserve. You will see that your energy envelope has broadened substantially. You will be able to do more in any day than you were able to do prior to initiating this activity program. And you'll find that you can do more without paying for it. Yes, you may have some setbacks. You may walk one day and have some worsening of your fatigue and pain. But on a three-day-a-week walking plan, you can always allow yourself an occasional "bad" day when you don't walk.

The bottom line: if you keep at it, your ability to tolerate activity will increase, and your actual amount of activity will increase too. And even more importantly, you will start feeling in control. Each of these is a step to wellness, and a step away from the deconditioning of your body that came from months or even years of inactivity. The symptoms of deconditioning will disappear, and with them your tendency to focus on your symptoms instead of on the positive aspects of your life. You'll be less afraid of activity because you'll begin to see it as a tool toward wellness, not a hindrance that will always set you back.

## If You Think All This Is Impossible

If you've read to this point but your current level of energy makes this wellness plan sound like pie in the sky, please don't become discouraged. I know from years of experience with hundreds of patients that you may think you'll *never* again regain the kind of energy that would enable you to walk as far as your driveway. Just getting out of bed may seem to demand all the energy you can muster right now. You're not alone, and your feelings are very real and entirely understandable. I'm just asking you to suspend disbelief and imagine for a moment that you can conserve all your energy to make that first, very short, very slow walk. Once you've done that, you'll be only at the beginning of your road to wellness. But that's better than not being on the road at all. Commit to wellness and you will succeed.

Everything I've mentioned here is a step-by-step roadmap to wellness. I've provided it in case you need to get yourself onto this road all by yourself. But finding a coach will help immeasurably. I mentioned the coach concept earlier in this chapter when I discussed cognitive behavioral therapy (CBT). Just who should this coach be? Let me start out with some don'ts: Don't pick a trainer and don't go to a physical therapist. Although people in these occupations are experts at helping people improve their fitness, they rarely have experience in dealing with people who have serious problems with fatigue or widespread bodily pain. They push too hard, often with disastrous results. Thus their weekly exercise prescription will almost definitely produce the yo-yo effect. And that is something to avoid.

In my own practice, I work with a wellness counselor who is an expert at coaching people to get on and stay on the road to wellness. Early on, while people are learning about their own energy capacity and daily expenditure, I recommend that they meet with the wellness counselor every two to three weeks. In effect, she acts as the person's buddy in designing the energy envelope, and then provides feedback in the earliest stages of moving along the road to wellness. So the goal is to find this kind of wellness counselor.

The most practical way to do this is to turn to CBT. But not just any cognitive behavioral therapist will be right for you. The best one will be a psychologist with complete training in CBT as well as experience in dealing with medically ill patients. Depending on where you live, your local pain management center (which may be freestanding or part of a hospital or clinic) is an excellent place to find such a counselor. If you can't find a pain management center, visit www.academyofct.org or www.nacbt.org, which provide a list of people who have gone through formal training to do this work. Before making an appointment, ask the person about his or her experience at dealing with people with chronic medical illness. You will need a person with that expertise to serve as your personal coach to wellness.

Why invest in CBT? Because unless you are an exceptionally self-motivated person, you will need someone to help you get on and stay on the wellness road. This means that you will need a guide to help you through the thicket of dealing with uncertainty. Unfortunately, doctors are not reimbursed purely on the basis of the time we spend talking with patients. That's too bad, because it means that doctors will not make this aspect of patient care part of their practice. But finding another professional who can be your guide on the road to wellness will be worth the effort.

# PART THREE

# WHAT ELSE YOU
# NEED TO KNOW

# 9

# Complementary Treatments

L et me lay out the golden rule of academic medicine. Researchers work on developing treatments, eliminating the myriad possibilities that either don't work or have more negative than positive effects. Finally, after arduous and expensive clinical testing for efficacy, the drug company submits its drug to the Food and Drug Administration (FDA) for approval. Only then does research turn into practice. We call this evidence-based medicine.

But as the last two chapters show, there are not that many treatments available for chronic fatigue syndrome (CFS), fibromyalgia (FM), and the other illnesses we've been discussing. So how can I promise to help every patient who walks into my office? I have my own golden rule that trumps the golden rule of medicine: I can *always* do something to help, so I *never* tell a patient the situation is hopeless. Traditional Western medical techniques fall under the heading of allopathic medicine, and serve us well as far as they go. But when they fall short, I try treatments some physicians would never think of trying—as long as they're safe. These methods aren't routinely taught to medical students, but they seem to help some people feel better. I view them as complementary to my usual medical approach.

But let me be clear: I have a set of rules for trying these treatments. Those rules are relatively simple, but they are still rules.

The premise for using these nontraditional treatments has to be rational and based on logic—or better yet, actual evidence—rather than simply on intuition. The treatment cannot be dangerous, and it cannot bankrupt the patient.

To these rules, I add the Natelson Six-Week Rule: I give a treatment six weeks to show that it helps. If after six weeks, the person isn't sure whether the treatment worked, I stop it. Discipline and medical common sense require that there be minimal uncertainty as to a treatment's efficacy, especially when drugs are involved. That prevents what I call the wheelbarrow phenomenon. My office asks new patients to bring all their medicines in, whether prescription based or not. Sad but true, too often the patient has accumulated so many medications over time that he or she practically needs a wheelbarrow to bring them to my office. It's no longer clear which of these drugs work and which don't. Very often we find they were prescribed by multiple physicians and specialists, or, in the case of food supplements or over-the-counter products, by no one at all.

The wheelbarrow goes beyond drugs. People who have been sick for a long time are apt to become more and more desperate in seeking help. When doctors tell such patients there's nothing wrong with them (and show them to the door without helping), they feel they have no alternative but to seek alternative treatments on their own. Since patients can't prescribe drugs for themselves, they often turn to an endless procession of nutritional supplements.

I'm still surprised by patients' automatic trust in these "natural" products. I sometimes find that when I *do* prescribe a drug, a patient making a return visit will tell me that he or she didn't try it, afraid of the side effects. But paradoxically, the patient will also tell me that he or she is taking a series of nutritional supplements or other products from the health-food store, without ever questioning the effects they may be causing. No matter where they were purchased, these products can have significant side effects of their own, either directly or by influencing how well actual drugs work. Just because they're "natural" does not mean using them carries no risk.

Need proof? Arsenic is a chemical element found in nature. It was used therapeutically in high doses in the eighteenth century, but today we know it to be a deadly poison. I'm not against novel, alternative treatments; as I said, I use them in my own treatment programs. But my first rule is to be cautious. Today's nutritional supplement could prove to be tomorrow's arsenic. Statistics maintained by the American Association of Poison Control Centers make this point and are scary. The number of poisonings from herbs, vitamins, and other dietary supplements increased nine-fold from 1983 to 2005. Of the 125,600 incidents reported that year, 27 ended in death. Even more worrisome is an FDA consultant's estimate that for every serious adverse event that is reported, 99 other serious events are not.

How can you be cautious? You can speak with your doctor. When doctors ask patients about medicines, the patient often assumes the doctor means prescription medicines. That's only part of the story. I want to know about all of the medicines and supplements my patients are taking and how much of each: prescriptive, over-the-counter, herbs, or something from the health-food store. Everything. That way I get an accurate index. When your doctor asks you about medicines, tell him or her about everything you take in the hope of improving your health.

## The Case for and against Nutraceuticals

We've all heard a lot lately about nutraceuticals. These naturally occurring chemicals are a part of our food but in addition to having nutritional value, they can influence how we feel. One well-known example is St. John's wort. While a number of early studies showed a positive effect of this nutraceutical in reducing symptoms of depression, a carefully controlled study sponsored by the National Institutes of Health (NIH) came up negative. So whether this food supplement is helpful in relieving depression is still up in the air. Nevertheless, consumers often buy it in an effort to try to help themselves.

These results lead to several immediate questions. Are nutraceuticals safe? Do they do what they say they'll do? While the standard of proof set by the FDA is high for pharmaceuticals, it is quite low for nutraceuticals. As long as a company can show that the product derives from food we would normally eat, it doesn't have to prove much else—as long as it doesn't claim the substance "cures," "mitigates," "treats," or "prevents" any specific illness. Talking about improving how the user "feels" or "functions" is perfectly fine. So actual therapeutic efficacy is not required for these substances to be on the market.

Some nutraceuticals have been tested a great deal; others, practically not at all. Let's look first at those nutraceuticals with a stronger scientific basis. A whole set of studies has focused on carnitine, a building block of life (an amino acid) that permits muscles to work normally. Carnitine is in food but it is also made within the body. Since carnitine plays an important role in muscle function, it is reasonable to check whether levels are low in people with medically unexplained fatigue and pain. And, in fact, some evidence exists that carnitine is low in people with these symptoms. Carnitine may be working in the brain rather than in the muscle. One elegant study showed that acetylcarnitine, another form of carnitine, was found in low levels in a number of brain regions. Moreover, an unblinded trial of carnitine was reported to produce symptom improvement in CFS.

Earlier, I described how double-blind drug trials, in which neither the patient nor the scientist knows who is receiving the real drug and who is taking a placebo, are the most accurate. We did our own double-blind placebo-controlled trial of Enerdyn, an Italian-made product containing proprionyl carnitine (a substance similar to acetylcarnitine). This nutraceutical also contains amounts of a vitaminlike substance called NADH, which was reported to improve CFS symptoms. If the claims about carnitine were right, it should have had a beneficial effect in chronic fatigue patients—and adding NADH to the Enerdyn preparation should have made it even more potent. But we found no evidence for improvement in the group taking the Enerdyn. They did no better than the group taking the placebo.

We had done an earlier study of a nutraceutical called Ambrotose and also found it to be ineffective in relieving symptoms of fatigue, poor sleep, and widespread pain. Another recent double-blind study of vitamins and antioxidants done in Europe also proved ineffective. These studies are important to consider because many people move to alternative medical treatments when classical medicine is not terribly helpful. I will discuss the tendency for you to do this and its consequences in more depth in the next chapter. But this brief review should raise a red flag for you. While the idea that a "natural" product may hold the answer for symptom relief in CFS, FM, or irritable bowel syndrome (IBS) may seem attractive, the few carefully done studies don't support your spending money to try them. And because these products are not under tight governmental control as is the case for drugs, they may have unknown, dangerous adverse effects.

Drugs can go through careful placebo-controlled double-blind trials and achieve positive results. But positive results don't always stand up to time and experience—especially if they are not based on large numbers of patients. And that's precisely why I turn to the Natelson Six-Week Rule. Even if a study seems carefully done and the product is neither expensive nor dangerous, sometimes it fails to survive the Natelson Six-Week Rule. Tested or not, I will then cease to use it with patients.

What are some examples? I can think of six reported to help CFS: *evening primrose oil*, a source of essential fatty acids necessary for building cells; a critical substance made in the body called *SAMe* (short for S-Adenosyl-Methionine), which was found to have a possible positive effect on depression but is quite expensive; intramuscular injections of *magnesium* to treat low red blood cell magnesium (besides not working, the shots hurt like the dickens); the vitaminlike substance called NADH that I mentioned earlier, which influences how cells work; and supplements of an adrenal hormone called *dehydroepiandrosterone* (DHEA), thought by some (but with little support for this stance) to be lacking in patients with the "invisible illnesses."

For a fact to be believed or a treatment to really work, more than one research team must show the same results; this process is called replication. And as a physician treating patients, I *still* apply one more obvious criterion: the treatment has to actually work in my patients, without causing any harm. I have tried each of the six treatments just mentioned but without any appreciable success.

In sum, the same caution that applies in using mainstream treatments also applies in using complementary or alternative ones, and even more so. But all of that said, the good news is that several complementary treatments *are* effective in reducing symptoms in people with medically unexplained illnesses. Let's look at them next, keeping in mind that there's more to alternative treatments than drugs and nutritional supplements. We've already seen how exercise and sleep can play roles in improving your health. In the sections that follow, we'll look at additional treatments, ranging from massage to yoga to changes in the diet and even tai chi.

## Alternative Treatments for Pain

People often ask me about three very common alternative treatments for pain: acupuncture, hypnosis, and massage. Three well-controlled studies have evaluated *acupuncture* in FM, and two of them reported positive results in reducing symptoms. One of these studies noted that fatigue was the symptom most improved, but that improvement tended to wane over time. In contrast, another study done on women with neck and shoulder pain producing headaches found improvement lasting several years. These studies were beautifully done in that the patients could not tell whether they were actually receiving acupuncture or not. These studies certainly encourage a trial of acupuncture for CFS, FM, or IBS pain. The nice thing about this course of treatment is that it fits within my Six-Week Rule. You will know by that time whether it works for you.

*Hypnotherapy* is another potentially useful technique with data suggesting its efficacy in reducing pain. One recent paper reported that hypnotherapy was initially helpful to a large group of patients with IBS; and, importantly, many of them maintained their improvement over time. Just how hypnosis actually works in IBS is a question for further research, but it is known to be useful for other kinds of pain too. So it should be able to help patients with FM as well as those with IBS.

Patients often report that massage helps relieve their pain. A physician at our local rehabilitation center got me interested in one particular form of massage known as *Rolfing* or *structural integration*. The theory behind this form of massage is that stress or injury displaces muscles and ligaments, causing other parts of the body to compensate. With prolonged compensation over time, the displacement becomes semipermanent. The idea of the treatment is to use deep massage to return these pathological states to normal. Because of the nature of the treatment, I call it *deep fibromuscular massage* or *release*.

The massage practitioner asks the person to walk, or else directly examines the muscles and joints, and is trained to see changes in motion of the body and thus to identify areas of restriction amenable to treatment. Treatment consists of ten sessions lasting about an hour each. While some patients with severe FM cannot tolerate this treatment—because it does stretch muscles and ligaments and can be quite painful—others report reduced pain and improved function afterward. This rather common outcome plus the fact that the treatment is relatively short in duration leads me to prescribe it for widespread pain. But I do this keeping two thoughts in mind. First, just because the treatment works does not mean that it does so because of the theories behind structural integration, and second, I don't know if this type of massage is any better than other methods of massage. What we have done is a very preliminary uncontrolled trial, and I have already explained to you why such results might disappear in a carefully done controlled trial. But the bottom line is that the treatment can help, and some of my patients swear by its use.

## Improving Balance and Wellness in Severe Fatigue

As a neurologist, part of my assessment of any new patient is a careful evaluation of his or her brain and nerve function. Fatigue can be a symptom of neurological disease, so I evaluate patients carefully for diseases such as multiple sclerosis that can cause fatigue. My basic rule is to confine the diagnosis of CFS to only those patients who have a normal neurological examination. But I will allow one abnormality: a minimal problem with balance. I do this because I do not believe that such a problem could in any way produce the kind of symptoms so common in my patients. I test balance by asking a patient to walk heel to toe, the way a police officer would test a suspected drunk driver for high levels of blood alcohol. In addition, I ask patients to maintain the heel-to-toe posture for a five-second period without moving and with their eyes closed. I would estimate that more than 10 percent of my patients have trouble with either of these tests.

That brought up an important question. Could I find objective evidence for these balance problems in CFS patients compared to people without CFS? To get answers, we used a computerized platform, which tilts back and forth while the patient tries to maintain balance, and found objective evidence that CFS patients do, indeed, experience more balance problems than other people. This is important because it is further evidence for our belief that some people experience severe fatigue due to some aberrancy of brain function.

Because some of our patients undergoing deep fibromuscular massage said they felt better overall and had less pain, my colleague, an expert in physical medicine, hypothesized that the treatment might improve the balance of CFS and FM patients. So he and another colleague, who was an expert in clinical research, tested patients' balance before and after they completed their course of massage treatment. To provide a comparison, they also tested untreated CFS and FM patients and healthy people on two occasions separated by several weeks.

If massage improved balance, we would expect to find better balance scores on the second trial than on the first. Since the comparison groups had no specific treatment between their two balance tests, we would expect similar scores on the two tests. The graph on page 193 shows the data. The dashed line going from the lower left to the upper right of the plot depicts the values that would be the same on the two balance tests. If balance did not improve, symbols representing each individual patient should lie on or near the dashed line. If balance did improve on the second trial, symbols should be above the dashed line. The data show that we found what we had expected. The normal volunteers and the untreated patients have results on the two test sessions that tend to lie on or along the

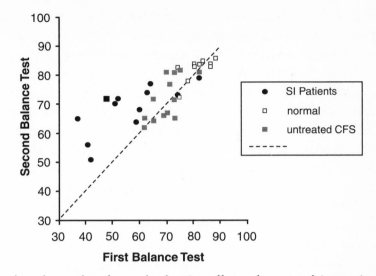

This graph plots the results of a study showing effects of structural integration massage on balance in CFS and FM patients compared to the untreated patients and normal controls.

dashed line. In contrast, patients undergoing the structural integration massage tended to have their points shifted up from the dashed line. So the data shows little or no change over time for healthy or sick people not given the massage treatment but improved balance for patients given the treatment. Moreover, the effect of the treatment was greatest for those people whose scores had started off the worst. After the massage intervention, they were the people who showed the greatest improvement in balance. And coincident with the improved balance, treated people reported having less pain.

The results of this study answer some questions and leave others unanswered, which is typical in research. For example, we know about the improvements, but we don't know why both balance and state of health improved with the massage. We also don't know what it was about the massage that led to these improvements. One possibility is that something related to muscle tightness or soreness interfered with the brain's control of balance, and that massage relieved this impasse. If so, it may have led to improved brain function, and that may have brought about improvements both in balance and the patients' overall feeling states. Answering these questions will take clever thinking with good experimental planning.

These preliminary data are quite encouraging, and our group is currently working on an application for federal funding to allow a more formal study on the effect of Rolfing on fatigue and pain. But until we can do such a study, I do think a trial of this type of massage is worth doing for anyone with deep muscle tenderness and balance problems. You will probably have a good idea as to whether you have a balance problem just based on your abilities to move around your home and outside environments. But if you want to confirm this, just try my heel-toe balance test with your eyes closed. If you are in this group, you can probably get a referral to a physical therapist or massage therapist who knows this technique, and your insurance will probably cover the treatment.

I'm giving balance particular attention because of our preliminary results. I don't know yet if other massage-related treatments besides fibromuscular massage improve balance and wellness, but my guess is that they might. That may be one reason why some of my patients with pain often report being helped by chiropractic massage and manipulation. Once again, applying the Natelson Six-Week Rule is important. If you see a benefit after six weeks, you and your doctor should discuss continuing the massage treatments. If you honestly haven't seen any results after six weeks, it will be time to move on to other treatments.

## Tai Chi

Another way to improve balance is to try *tai chi*, an ancient Chinese martial art that has become popular in this country as an exercise and relaxation technique. I mentioned this form of gentle exercise in chapter 6 as a way of reducing stress. Before I developed the walking regimen that I laid out in chapter 8, I had used tai chi to get people started increasing their activity. My current use of this exercise is for people with balance problems on the neurological exam. Although tai chi has never been formally tested in medically unexplained illness, a number of studies have shown that it improves balance and stability. Given the positive results we've seen from fibromuscular massage, I'm willing to try a safe technique that improves balance, may reduce other symptoms, and may also improve a person's overall well being. For individuals who cannot gain access to fibromuscular massage, tai chi is an appropriate alternative. Even if you can't find a tai chi class in your area, you'll certainly be able to learn the basics from books.

### Vibration

Finally there is a new experimental way of improving balance. This method uses a new concept in neurological research—that marginally effective parts of the nervous system will work better if the connections to them are enhanced by stimulation from an outside source. Using a similar balance testing device to the moving platform I've already mentioned, Dr. Jim Collins was able to improve the relatively poor balance of elderly people by having them stand on vibrating inner soles. The vibration was transmitted through peripheral nerves into the brain to augment the activity of its balance center. Dr. Collins is developing a version of these inner soles that may soon become available in stores.

## Improving Breathing to Reduce Stress

The last chapter in this book will answer the question that every one of my patients asks, "What's new [in CFS, FM, IBS research]?" But one of these novel areas of research can't wait until then. The story began with a report that patients with medically unexplained fatigue and pain developed very low blood pressure and fainting during a postural challenge—lying on a table that tilted up. This result received a great deal of attention in the national media, because it suggested that patients with CFS or FM had a disease of the nerves to their heart and blood vessels. The publicity about this delayed neurogenic hypotension was such that many patients went to their doctor asking to get tilt testing.

As I have explained, science advances when important results can be replicated by other people in other laboratories. Several groups, including our own, tried to duplicate the tilt-testing result but came up empty-handed. We had two explanations for the discrepancy. First, the original study required subjects to have an intravenous needle in place; it is well known that puncturing the skin predisposes people to fainting. And second, subjects in the original study—but not in our own—might have been taking low doses of drugs that could affect transmission of nerve impulses to the blood vessels. But not all of the results have been negative. A colleague of mine at New York Medical College has replicated these results in unmedicated children and adolescents with CFS. To me, this suggests that CFS behaves differently in kids from how it does in adults.

Regardless, these experiments focused my attention on the common complaint that patients with CFS or FM often feel worse while standing than they do when lying down. While delayed drops in blood pressure did not seem to be a problem after all, dramatic increases in heart rate when standing did seem to be an issue, and one seen in some patients with CFS. This sensitivity to standing manifested by an increase in heart rate is called *postural orthostatic tachycardia syndrome* (POTS). The causes of POTS will be discussed in chapter 11.

Because of the existence of POTS in some CFS patients, and because many of my own CFS patients say they feel much worse while standing, I did a preliminary or pilot study that extended our biological measurements to include breathing as well as cardiovascular function during a simple postural challenge. I asked my patients to start by lying quietly in the supine position. In that position, I counted heart and breathing rates, measured blood pressure, and also measured the amount of carbon dioxide exhaled with each breath. There is very little carbon dioxide in air; it is made in the body when foods are burned with oxygen. The carbon dioxide goes from the blood into the lungs, where it is excreted with each breath, and levels fall to very low values when a person hyperventilates.

Each of these measures has a range that is considered normal: heart rate from about 60 to about 85; blood pressure from about 100 over 60 to just under 140 over 90; breathing rate per minute from about 10 to 18; and exhaled carbon dioxide from 36 to 44. Then I continued doing these measurements every minute for eight minutes with the person standing while leaning against a wall and not moving.

I found surprising results in the sixty-two patients I studied. More than half had some abnormality. Although I expected to find a lot of POTS, I found it in a minority—in only five of the thirty-two patients with abnormalities. But the biggest group was one I hadn't previously identified: thirteen of my patients had what I am calling *postural orthostatic syndrome of hyperventilation* (POSH). While lying down, these patients breathed normally; but when they stood, they breathed more than necessary, and so their exhaled carbon dioxide levels fell to 30 or below. This marked change in breathing with resulting low levels of carbon dioxide in the blood is probably responsible for some patients feeling awful when they stand for prolonged periods of time. I am currently working on experiments to understand the why of this important finding.

In addition, I found that two patients hyperventilated—breathed more than was necessary—both while lying quietly in the supine position and while standing. This overbreathing reduced their blood levels of carbon dioxide to low levels that are associated with symptoms including severe fatigue, achiness, dizziness, and numbness in the fingers and toes and around the lips. Early work trying to understand the cause of chronic fatigue syndrome suggested that it was due to chronic hyperventilation through most of the waking day. This pilot study shows that this result can happen but not frequently. So chronic hyperventilation may be one cause of CFS, but certainly not a common one.

It's still worth while, however, to consider whether chronic hyperventilation is a factor for you. If you want to test yourself for hyperventilation, you can do so quite easily. Use a watch to determine how long you can hold your breath after you breathe in deeply. Most people can hold their breath for about forty-five seconds. If you can hold your breath for only thirty-five seconds or less, you may have this breathing problem. To determine whether you might have POSH, stand up straight without moving for at least eight minutes. If you feel ill while standing, you might have "orthostatic intolerance," which could be due to

POSH. To check this out, repeat the standing test later, this time breathing into a paper bag held across your nose and mouth. (Don't use a plastic bag, which could be dangerous.) The paper bag acts as a reservoir for carbon dioxide, preventing you from blowing off too much. If you are more comfortable standing while you breathe into the bag, this is pretty good evidence that you are blowing off too much carbon dioxide and that you have POSH.

Whether hyperventilation or POSH is the diagnosis for you, you may be able to use *breathing retraining* to lessen your symptoms and feel better. The way you breathe influences the autonomic nervous system, or ANS—the nerves that connect the brain to the heart, blood vessels, and the gut. When your body is preparing for action, your heart rate and blood pressure go up, while digestion stops. Later, when calm returns, your heart rate and blood pressure return to normal, and digestion resumes. So there are two parts of the ANS—one to prepare for action and the other to prepare for relaxation. Good health requires a balanced ANS. If the ANS is not properly balanced, you can experience diarrhea, constipation, abdominal pain, and fatigue. Moreover, changes in ANS balance can produce POTS as well as a sudden decrease in blood pressure when you are standing.

## The Autonomic Nervous System

One major factor in producing autonomic imbalance is stress. We don't know all the ways that stress alters the autonomic nervous system, but we do know that one mechanism is by changing the way you breathe. There is a natural coupling between healthy breathing and the time between individual heart beats. If you breathe into your belly, slowly and completely, the speed of each beat of your heart varies considerably as you breathe in and out. If your breathing is rapid and irregular, and if you don't completely expand and empty your lungs, variability between beats disappears, and your heart beats like a metronome. In general, breathing from your abdomen or belly is healthier than breathing from high in your chest. Chest breathing consumes energy and is inefficient. Abdominal, belly, or diaphragmatic breathing *is* efficient and will help you stop overbreathing. Naturally enough, the variability between heart beats is called *heart rate variability*, and higher levels of this breathing-related variability are associated with a more balanced ANS and better health. In short, deep breaths are better than shallow ones, and a variable heart rate is healthier than a completely regular one. By retraining the way you breathe, you can rebalance your ANS. This should help you feel less stressed—and help you stand up longer without feeling awful.

It can be very instructive to check on your breathing habits in this way, and if you find an abnormality you'll actually have learned something potentially very positive. And simply being aware of what is happening can be reassuring. You will understand that some of your most uncomfortable feelings of pain or fatigue may be caused by a breathing problem you can easily treat, not by some horrible disease. If stress is a problem for you or if this chapter has helped you identify breathing as a possible problem, ask your doctor to send you for physical or respiratory therapy. Some but not all physical therapists or respiratory therapists are knowledgeable about how to help you change the way you breathe.

The important thing to emphasize here is that breathing retraining works and can help you feel a lot better, so commit to doing it. If you choose not to go to your doctor, here are two self-help methods to try. The first method uses *biofeedback*, a technique mentioned in chapter 6. Biofeedback means that you can alter your biology if you can see it in action and practice making it go in a direction associated with feeling better. Many biofeedback therapists do work on helping people learn new ways to breathe, but few use the special equipment needed to measure levels of exhaled carbon dioxide. Since devices to do this have been expensive until recently, appreciation of breathing pattern disorders by both doctors and psychologists is not as high as it should be, and so this cause of symptoms often goes unrecognized.

Additionally, not all biofeedback therapists have experience with breathing retraining, since most patients referred to this therapy suffer from migraine headaches. Biofeedback therapists reduce stress—and thus the risk of migraine—by teaching people to use the ANS to relax and dilate (enlarge) their blood vessels, usually in the fingertip. They know this has happened when the temperature in the fingertip increases, which shows that more blood is reaching this extremity. Since the ANS is also involved in breathing, you can see how the same mechanisms might be used to help people improve their breathing techniques. In fact, biofeedback experts can now use a computer program supplied with a heart rate sensor called *Freeze-Framer* to track breathing indirectly, based on the relation between breathing and heart rate variability—the tighter the link, the lower the stress level. There will be further discussions on this link in chapter 11. But it's useful to know that advances in computer technology have brought the cost of the Freeze-Framer down from thousands of dollars to $275 on the Internet—still a lot, but a big improvement. This form of biofeedback may thus be within your reach to try at home, whereas just a few years ago only a handful of specialists could have afforded it. And besides reducing overbreathing and stress, my colleague Dr. Paul Lehrer tells me that use of a method similar to Freeze-Framer was effective in reducing pain and improving function in FM patients.

Freeze-Framer gives you an overall look at how well your breathing is linked to your heart rate. In addition to the display of your heart rate over time, it gives you an accumulated coherence score. As the link between your heart and your breathing continues to improve, your coherence will go up, and the program will tell you that you are in *the zone*. This indicates good coupling between heart rate and breathing, a state in which stress begins to disappear. Twice-daily breathing practice using the Freeze-Framer device can help you employ healthier breathing. After a week or two of practice, you may be able to do this breathing exercise at the highest skill level in the program or even without the biofeedback provided by the Freeze-Framer program. That means that you can adapt this breathing strategy when you feel the first biological manifestations of stress or if you feel uncomfortable while standing. Do a Web search for Freeze-Framer to learn about the program and get this tool for the best price. I provide detail on its use not available in the instruction manual in an appendix at the end of this book. A portable version not requiring a computer became available in the spring of 2007.

## Special Yogic Breathing Exercises

A second strategy for retraining breathing (and thus reducing stress) uses a form of yoga in which breathing exercises are emphasized over more demanding physical body movements—Kundalini yoga (KY). In chapter 6, I mentioned Hatha yoga as a technique for reducing stress. However, Hatha yoga requires considerable amounts of energy and often proves difficult for people with severe fatigue or pain. In contrast, KY is less physically demanding. There really aren't any data on the efficacy of these breathing exercises in improving fatigue, but healthy breathing means good ANS balance with fewer symptoms and, ultimately, less stress. In addition, they are simple and cost nothing. Despite the lack of scientific data, people have done these exercises for many hundreds of years. It seems reasonable to me to assume that people have done these yogic practices over the years because the exercises made them feel better.

Kundalini yoga is based on a Hindu understanding about the way the body is organized. Quite frankly, though, I'm less concerned with the theory and philosophy underlying these exercises than with their medical effects, and I encourage my patients with breathing problems to give these exercises a try. Some of the exercises designed to get you into a relaxed state require you to say or chant a few phrases. This is called a mantra. Chapter 6 noted that Dr. Herbert Benson dispensed with these in teaching people a simplified way to meditate. However, the teachers of this form of yoga are pretty adamant that the sound you make when you say or chant the mantra can be health enhancing. So why not chant the mantra?

David Shanahoff-Khalsa, a researcher studying how these breathing exercises affect the body and an expert in KY, introduced me to this form of yoga. There are a huge number of possible exercises to do. I asked David to suggest a few specifically aimed at reducing fatigue. I haven't given you all the ones he suggested because I believe in starting low and going slow. Do the following sample exercises only once a day.

*The tuning-in exercise.* The purpose of this first exercise is to relax you and to prepare your entire body for the subsequent exercises.

Sit in a chair with a straight spine and with your feet flat on the floor. Put your hands together at the chest in prayer pose, pressing the palms together with a medium amount of pressure. The area where the sides of the thumbs touch rests on your sternum or ribcage, with the thumbs pointing up, and you should keep your fingers together and pointing up and out, at a sixty-degree angle to the ground. Close your eyes, but focus as if you're looking off into the distance. Inhale first through your nose and chant "Ong Namo," with an equal emphasis on "Ong" and "Namo." Then immediately follow with a half-breath inhalation through the mouth and chant "Guru Dev Namo," again with approximately equal emphasis on each word. The sound you generate is thought to help you relax. (The easiest way to learn the rhythm of this mantra is to hear it chanted by an expert, which you can do on the Internet at the Web site www.kundaliniyoga .net/fy1.htm.) Repeat this breathing cycle at least three times and then stop. Do this once a day for a sufficient amount of time that you are comfortable with this exercise. Then over the next two weeks, increase the number of repetitions from three to ten.

*Spine flexing for vitality.* Avoid eating just before doing this exercise. Sit in a chair, holding your knees with both hands for support and leverage. Pull the chest up and forward, inhaling deeply at the same time. Then relax the spine into a slouching position as you exhale. Breathe both in and out through your nose. To prevent a whip action of your neck, try not to let your head move much with the flexing action of the spine. Start slowly to loosen up your spine—one cycle every 2 to 3 seconds. Close your eyes and concentrate on the sound of the breathing. If your mind wanders, try to bring it back to focus on your breathing. Do this for 1 minute at first, gradually increasing over time to 2 minutes. Then over the next several weeks, pick up the speed at which you do these exercises until you can do one cycle of spine extension and flexion in one second. Feel free to extend the duration of this exercise to up to 5 minutes. Should you feel light-headed, stop momentarily and then continue. Relax for 1 to 2 minutes when finished.

*Shoulder shrugs for vitality.* Sit with your spine straight, resting your hands on your knees. Inhale and raise your shoulders up toward your ears, then exhale, letting your shoulders down again. Breathe only through your nose; keep your eyes closed and focus into the distance. As before, listen to the sound of your inhalation and exhalation. If your mind wanders, try to bring it back to the sound of your breathing. Continue this action rapidly, building to three times per second for a maximum time of 2 minutes.

*Technique against fatigue and listlessness.* If you are pregnant or have high blood pressure, skip this exercise. Sit with a straight spine. Place the palms together as you did in the tuning-in exercise. Close your eyes, trying to look up to where your nose meets your eyebrows. As you inhale, break the breath into four equal parts, while counting one-two-three-four. Hold your breath for a few seconds and then exhale by again breaking the breath into four equal parts, again counting out loud. Then hold your breath for a few seconds before starting the cycle again. On each part of the inhale or exhale pull the navel point in slightly. One full cycle or breath takes about 7 to 8 seconds, and you should continue this pattern for 2 minutes. Then inhale deeply and press the palms together with medium force for 10 seconds. Relax for 15 to 30 seconds. Then repeat this entire procedure twice. When finished, if necessary, lie on your back with your eyes closed and relax your entire body for 2 minutes. As you become more comfortable doing this exercise, increase the force with which you press your palms together over a number of sessions, finally doing it with maximal force. Then increase the duration of the entire exercise to 3 to 5 minutes.

## Nutritional Issues

People always ask me whether changing their diet might help them feel better. The idea that you can greatly influence your health by taking food supplements or by altering your diet seems natural and is encouraged by the health food industry. There will be more to say about this industry in the next chapter. Changing what you eat, and how you eat it, doesn't necessarily mean buying a lot of expensive new products. And, indeed, there have been reports of health improvements following dietary manipulation. Much of the research on the effects of diet on rheumatological diseases, including FM, comes from Scandinavia. A number of trials have shown some success in reducing symptoms and signs of inflammation in rheumatoid arthritis following limited periods of fasting and with subsequent strict dietary restriction. Similarly, being on a strict vegan diet for three months led to improved sleep and less pain in a group of FM patients. The diet used is called *the living food diet*: all food is served uncooked and consists of fruit, berries, vegetables, mushrooms, nuts, seeds, legumes, and cereals.

With such a diet, vitamin supplements are a must. Diets such as these are usually less than 2,000 calories per day and so lead to weight loss—a side benefit. On the other hand, your body can't get all of the vital nutrients it needs from fruits and vegetables alone, so this diet can be dangerous; that's the reason vitamin supplements are critical. As you can see, this is a very strict diet that you may decide is not terribly practical even to consider. The bottom line is that these diets can help, but they are very demanding and in this regard not terribly practical. But if you are interested in trying one of these, I would recommend that you do so in close consultation with a nutritionist.

Even if symptoms are not improved by these diets, they do accomplish one thing—weight loss, and for many that result is desirable and empowering because you put yourself in control and did it. I also use a diet as part my therapeutic approach, but one that is easier to follow and better balanced than these exclusion diets. In coming up with my own diet plan, I have opted for the sensible rather than the dramatic.

## The Natelson Diet

Weight gain is a problem for many people with medically unexplained illness. Some of this is a side effect of being less active than previously. Sometimes it is a side effect of treatment for depression. The selective serotonin reuptake inhibitors (SSRIs) and the tricyclic antidepressants (TCAs) are notorious for causing weight gain. Prior to the release of duloxetine onto the market, I usually initiated my pain management program with low doses of the TCAs and still do so when finances are an issue. Even though these medicines do help, even at low dosages they can promote a weight gain so bothersome that some patients will stop taking them. This seems to be less of a problem when I start my pain management regimen with duloxetine (see chapter 7 for details).

However, weight gain remains an issue for the majority of my patients who are taking antidepressants and have had to greatly reduce their physical activity because of fatigue or pain. A major way to combat this is the program for gentle aerobic conditioning that I laid out in detail in the last chapter. The Natelson diet is the second arm of this treatment.

Exercise and diet lead to weight loss. Although the craze seems to be fading now, in recent years much of the United States was swept away by the high-fat, low-carbohydrate diet fad. Even though cholesterol and other cardiovascular risk factors actually improve on this diet in the short term, I still have concerns about its emphasis on ingesting a lot of fat. My diet is still low on carbohydrates, but I've taken care to balance increases in fat intake with increases in protein intake. I like to call it the "healthy Atkins diet"—in contrast to the less-healthy original—so don't expect to see me recommending that you eat tons of butter and bacon. I have to hasten to say that I have not done any controlled studies on the efficacy of the Natelson diet, but my patients do lose weight on this diet, and then find it easier to do the walking exercises I recommended earlier—as well as feel better about themselves.

So please try this diet for three weeks. Why do I ask for three weeks instead of the six I require so much of the time? Any diet is hard to follow, because it means changing habits that may have been with you for many years. But I'm sure you'll agree with me that a three-week commitment is not much of a hardship, especially if you see results. The other nice thing about the diet is that it is another way to put you in control of yourself. As I've mentioned previously, illness is disempowering, and very often people feel that they've lost command of their own bodies. Here's a way to get back into control. If at the end of the three-week trial you have lost any weight, you should view that as a success—and worthy of extending the trial for another three weeks.

The basic idea is to move toward a simple elemental diet while restricting carbohydrates. The nice thing about this diet is that you can eat as much of the allowable foods as you want to fill up. By "elemental" I mean that you should eat foods without additives like food coloring or stabilizers. In fact, the only additives allowed are Nutrasweet or Splenda to substitute for whole sugar.

And you'll have to stay away from carbs altogether. I don't think it essential to have a workbook with a list of the carbohydrate counts in each food. A simpler way to avoid high-carb foods is to remember which general categories you should avoid completely. Stop consuming anything with alcohol in it (wine, beer, or liquor) and stop eating starchy foods like rice, potatoes, corn, bread, or cake. In fact, you should cut out desserts altogether for these three weeks—don't even think about buying the so-called low-carb desserts or supplements that are now filling the supermarket. For this diet to work, you really have to cut back on carbohydrates, not substitute one for another.

You should cut out fruits, too (they're loaded with sugar), and eat only green leafy vegetables—no beets or carrots, and no tomatoes or tomato products, such as ketchup. Plus, you should drink at least eight glasses of water a day. The fluids help prevent one of the common side effects of low-carbohydrate diets—constipation. Obviously, if you start out with constipation as a primary symptom, this diet is probably not for you.

I should say a bit more about beverages, because water—while unbeatable—can get pretty boring after a few days. Alternatives include homemade lemonade or a low-calorie version you can buy. Making your own lemonade isn't nearly as hard as you might imagine. Fill a glass with ice and seltzer water. (I prefer seltzer water to club soda because it is usually cheaper and has no added salt.) Hand-squeeze a quarter of a lemon or lime into the glass. Add some sweetener to your taste (Nutrasweet or Splenda—*not* sugar) and drink. You will have no trouble drinking eight glasses of either of these choices per day.

If possible, over the three-week trial, try to follow the food recommendations that I lay out next, which is simpler than trying to come up with alternatives each day. Breakfast may seem like a problem at first, since carb-laden breads and cereals are out; but here's a great substitute that's easy to prepare, and more interesting than toast anyway. Buy the cheapest version of Egg-Beaters that you can find. Essentially, this food product removes the cholesterol from eggs while leaving all the healthy parts behind. If your supermarket carries tofu products (look in the coolers in the produce aisle, or even the department that sells sliced cheese and meat products), you can liven up scrambled Egg-Beaters by adding tofu pepperoni (use two to three slices per plate) and tofu cheese slices (I prefer the pepper jack or cheddar with jalapeño). So breakfast consists of a scrambled Egg-Beater omelet with phony pepperoni and phony cheese. No fat and plenty of protein. The easiest way to make this dish is via the microwave. Cook the egg and pepperoni for 1 minute; then add the tofu cheese and microwave the dish for another 40 to 60 seconds, depending on the amount of Egg-Beaters you started with. For a change of pace, substitute pieces of smoked salmon or mushrooms instead of the pepperoni. This omelet, plus coffee or tea, is your breakfast. If you drink tea, choose green tea.

Lunch could consist of canned tuna fish or salmon with low-fat mayonnaise and cucumber slices on top of a slice of lettuce. For a change of pace, eat four to six slices of low-fat sliced cheese with mustard, or go with the tofu cheese. Use nuts as snacks if you get hungry between lunch and dinner. Dinner requires a bit more work in that you will have to prepare the main dish—either chicken, turkey, or fish. If you crave red meat, that's okay, but not more than once a week. Limiting red meat reduces your fat intake while still giving you a lot of protein.

Consider roasting a small turkey. You'll have plenty of leftovers for several lunches, either as slices to be eaten with mayonnaise or mustard or as turkey salad with mayonnaise, cucumbers, and onions. (Again, remember—no bread.) Vegetables with your dinner should consist of mushrooms, asparagus, broccoli, or green beans. No broad beans of any sort (lima, navy, Boston, or the like), which are starchy, and again no potatoes, corn, or rice. For those of you who don't want to have to think about just what to prepare, a good book that you can use to fill in the blanks about what to serve when is *The 30-Day Low-Carb Diet Solution* by Michael R. Eades, M.D., and Mary Dan Eades, M.D.

One supplement I do recommend when you are on the diet is a good once-a-day vitamin tablet. If your doctor is in agreement, perhaps he or she will prescribe Strohvite Advance. I prescribe this vitamin to patients with mild to moderate fatigue and to patients going onto my diet. It's a prescription vitamin usually used during pregnancy, so it is very complete. It's not gender-specific, so it's fine for men too.

Although you can switch from red meat to fowl and then to fish, you probably should try to stick with only one major food source for at least a week, allowing yourself red meat on the last day of the week. The simpler and more consistent your food intake is from day to day, the easier it will be to figure out if any of these food restrictions has an effect on your symptoms. Even if no single restriction makes you feel better, it's likely that the overall diet will; and as I said before, you'll also benefit from feeling that you've taken charge of your health again.

If you can combine this diet with a gentle aerobic conditioning regimen, that will improve the weight-loss results. Remember that one reason diets often seem to fail is that people continue to avoid exercise, even when they're capable of doing it. Reducing your caloric intake is great, but living a sedentary lifestyle makes your metabolism slow down. When that happens, weight gain is more common than weight loss, even if you *are* on a diet. So try to do some walking. Follow the regimen I laid out in chapter 8.

Here's another tip: Don't obsess over your scale. While you're on the diet, don't weigh yourself more often than once a week. Weighing yourself more often is practically a guarantee of disappointment, like watching a kettle come to a boil. You'll need to be on the diet for some days before you see any results, anyway. But if you find that you have lost weight after the three-week trial period, continue with the diet for at least another three weeks. Seeing pounds disappear over a six-week period should encourage you to continue for another six-week period. Your new eating habits will seem less strange by then—you may even find you've come to enjoy "cheese" made out of tofu. And if you have noticed any relief of your pain or fatigue, I urge you to stick with the diet a full three months, which is usually an adequate period to see real results.

Then, even if you add some carbohydrates back into your diet, you will probably continue to have the health benefits of the diet if you continue with the same elemental food outline, except now the diet will be well rounded. Feeling poorly about yourself because of weight gain is a negative that we can all do without. Losing weight on the Natelson diet is part of your toolbox for getting on the road to wellness.

# 10

# From Complementary Medicine to Quackery

I t's useful to draw lines between treatments that are beneficial, those that are not beneficial but are essentially harmless, and those that are not only useless but potentially harmful.

You already know that allopathic (or Western) medicine is beneficial, even though the treatments doctors prescribe often come with the bite of unwanted and potentially dangerous side effects. Despite this cost, traditional medicine's evidence-based progress over the decades has led to fantastic results. Americans live longer than ever before, and do so with a much higher quality of life than at any time in history. Better research and an ever-expanding arsenal of drugs has virtually eliminated diseases like polio and smallpox that once ruined or even ended lives, and terrified just about everybody.

The current focus of medicine is to use *high-tech* approaches to develop new drugs and medical procedures. Despite the benefit for patients, this approach leads to a problem: some of the *lower*-tech means of treating patients—the art of medicine that allows the doctor to hear the patient—fall by the wayside. This problem is due not only to high-tech ways of developing new medical treatments, but also to decisions about what medical insurance will cover, and for how much money. Unfortunately, an entire way of thinking about and relating to patients and their wellness has been a casualty of the new emphasis on high-tech and fast results.

The consequences of this focus have not hit yet, but they will. Medical schools will spend even more of medical students' time on teaching new mechanical procedures and techniques and less on teaching them how to hear you and understand how you feel and think. That will lead to more diagnoses of "nothing wrong"—even when something very definitely *is* wrong. Then people will again be left feeling that they're on their own when it comes to finding a pathway to wellness. But that's not to say that we should leave the evidence-based approach behind. Whatever its drawbacks, if combined with the low-tech "art of medicine" approach, the evidence-based approach is still the best at informing doctors about what medicine or procedure to use to relieve patient suffering.

In chapters 7, 8, and 9, I guided you through a series of possible therapeutic steps, some of them very definitely rooted in complementary medicine. Rejecting this broad-brush approach means that you will have to be your own doctor. I don't think that's ever a good choice. There's a difference between taking an active role in your care while working with professionals and imagining that you can do it all by yourself, deciding which treatment practices to choose and rely on. Too often, the do-it-yourself approach leads people down a slippery—and often costly—slope, toward medicines and treatments that are not supported by findings based on any scientific evidence. I call this approach "alternative," in that its methods are radically different from the broad-brush approach we've been discussing up to this point.

There's room in this approach for complementary techniques. These are techniques that are an adjunct to standard medical practice. For example, I might add acupuncture to my pharmacological pain management regimen, detailed in chapter 7. I go further than many doctors in trying complementary techniques like yoga and breathing exercises with my patients, and discussed many of these techniques in the last chapter. Many of these treatments grow out of non-Western medicine, a branch of medicine that is not so much evidence-based as it is time-tested. And I am sure that as Western medicine learns more about these techniques—and has the opportunity to test them further—still others will come into use. But in order to be adopted more widely, any treatment has to be shown to work—just as was done with acupuncture—by careful clinical trials looking at actual health outcomes.

## Alternative Medicine

There's a difference, then, between complementary medical techniques that can work alongside allopathic medicine even though they come from other traditions, and alternative medicine that turns its back on the traditional approach outright. Some examples would include the belief of some chiropractors that spinal manipulation can treat diseases such as asthma, or the idea of homeopathy that diluting a toxin a million-fold makes it able to relieve symptoms that are similar to those produced by the toxin. Some people believe there is an herb to treat every complaint. Your grandmother may have believed, as mine did, that chicken soup was the perfect cure for a fever. The way my grandmother's soup tasted, it sure couldn't hurt one way or the other, and it certainly was soothing and comforting. But even though some research has suggested that chicken soup does, indeed, have antiviral properties, it is *not* a valid first-line treatment for an infection. Giving up on allopathic medicine for any of these unproven alternatives just doesn't make sense.

Some of my patients tell me they feel better after taking supplements. The problem with such a testimonial is that it is from only one individual. While improvement is wonderful even for one person, you can't count on being number two. The FDA never allows a drug to come to market until it has been shown to work across large numbers of patients. The long wait for approval may seem frustrating or even cruel, but it's far better than the alternatives: allowing drugs with dangerous side effects to come to market or allowing patients to rely on drugs that cause improvement in few patients, or none. A few positive results, even if wonderful, don't count. Anyway, why should you accept the claims of those who purvey alternative treatments—with no proof—that their method works to the exclusion of all others? Let me be clear. I am not saying that alternative methods do not work. I *simply do not know* and am leery about your spending your money on unproven therapies.

After all, peddlers of alternative therapies may simply be trying to sell more of a product: not exactly a good reason to trust someone. And remember the issue of toxicity that I just mentioned. Traditional medicine has plenty to offer; you just have to find the right doctor.

Today, alternative treatments are legion. Magazine ads and Web sites offer testimonials about the efficacy of literally thousands of food products that *sound* as if they might be helpful. Be careful—more often than not, these seemingly heartfelt comments by "actual" users amount to little more than a high-pressure sales technique—one aimed specifically at people whose chronic illnesses have made them feel desperate. Especially when they have the added feeling that the medical system has bounced them around without really listening or caring, they may be all too susceptible and vulnerable to claims that a cure lies just around the corner, from a pill or a powder. If this promise were real, I would have no patients. But I have all too many.

## My Approach

So now you need to take personal account. If you've used the advice in this book to find a physician who really listens and works with you, then traditional allopathic medicine—plus my prescription for getting you on the path to wellness—can help you feel better. I view my job in helping you like painting by number. First, I fill in the threes and reduce some of your fatigue. Next, I fill in the ones and then the sevens, and you tell me that your pain is a bit less. After still another intervention, you may report that you are no longer depressed. I don't promise a cure, and you should be wary of anybody who does, particularly if that person has a product to sell. The operative word is *better*. I think my promising to make you better is very good when you remember that this promise doesn't hold for many diseases.

Moving to wellness is a slow process, and frustrating for that reason. The doctor alone cannot help you; you have to participate in wellness yourself. And this is not easy. The fact that all this is hard leads to the understandable desire for a faster and easier result—something you can take or do and get instantly better. But the solution isn't to move more quickly; it's to find a doctor who will be patient *with* you, and who will keep working with you to improve your health bit by bit. And it takes your own commitment to wellness.

An actively engaged relationship between you and your doctor can help you sort through the many available alternative therapies to find those that truly can be complementary to the other parts of your care. While I'm negative about therapies that make outrageous promises, I'm probably more accepting of nonallopathic approaches than many of my colleagues are. What's important, for me and for my patients, is that I work to understand their frustrations and their efforts to do things on their own. If one of my patients feels strongly about trying an alternative therapy, I lay out the risks as I see them. If I think the patient is taking a health risk with a therapeutic choice, I try hard to convince him or her not to try that treatment. If the risk is only to the pocketbook, I say to give it a try but to keep my rules in mind.

Is the treatment risky? The alternative practitioner is not the person to ask. You don't need your doctor's endorsement of the alternative treatment you are going to try, either—just his or her help in assessing the risk of that treatment. Then follow the Natelson Six-Week Rule. If you are confident that this treatment makes you feel better, continue. Maybe you are the one in a hundred for whom this treatment works or maybe the treatment would work on others if it were actually tested. If you feel the same or worse, *stop*. Remember that having these rules gives you some degree of control in a very cloudy area and gives you the perspective to move on if you're not sure whether you are better.

## The Modafinil Trial

Now, before going on, I need to make a point that may help make the rest of this discussion clearer. In chapter 7, I told you about the double-blind placebo-controlled trial we did in collaboration with four other sites for the antifatigue drug modafinil. I told you the results of the trial were negative in that we were unable to prove that the drug relieved fatigue. But then I told you that I continue to try it on patients anyway, which is contrary to the rules of evidence-based medicine I have tried to share with you throughout this book. I break my own rule for two reasons: I am quite positive the drug helps some people (this seemed to be the case for several of the smaller sites in the multicenter trial I headed), and modafinil happens to be a drug we can try within the standard of the Natelson Six-Week Rule. If it fails to have an effect, we'll know it within six weeks.

Modafinil is not like an antibiotic that is nearly uniformly successful in curing infection. Instead, its effect varies depending on the person, with only about a third reporting really good results. Since chronic fatigue, fibromyalgia, irritable bowel, and the other conditions we've been discussing are all syndromes, by definition they lump together illnesses with multiple causes. If that is the case, no drug will have a uniform result on everyone who tries it. The trick will be to design another trial that takes this variability into account. I hope to do this. Meanwhile, although I am bending my own rule a bit when I try modafinil with some patients, I do it only within narrow parameters, and with a definite therapeutic plan in mind. Doctors often conduct such "single-patient therapeutic trials" in their attempts to help their patients.

But what happens when you're on your own, trying an alternative medicine product without a doctor's guidance? The only expert you can rely on is the product's own manufacturer and the broad claims on the product label. Not only may these claims have no limits, but neither may the quantities of the product you're expected to buy before you'll see results. You may be taking a product for months only to find that it's had no positive effect. My advice is buyer beware. There are plenty of quacks out there.

## Quacks

The extreme definition of a quack is simple: someone who knowingly tries to defraud you into spending money with a false promise of either a cure or substantial relief, someone who makes a living selling the promise of wellness with products that couldn't possibly do anything. These are the snake-oil salesmen of the twenty-first century.

There are knowing charlatans, but there are also people who are true believers in the treatments they espouse, even though those treatments may be totally ineffective. They may latch onto an idea that makes sense to them and try it on a few patients. Because of their belief in their idea, they may think it works even when it doesn't. Sometimes their profound belief in the treatment is so persuasive that the placebo effect takes over, and the patient actually believes there have been positive results. Would that the medical profession could bottle this effect.

So, consider the practitioner who has a treatment guaranteed to cure you; the physician who charges you $5,000 for an evaluation and then sells you a product that he or she endorses (and may even make); or the physician who listens to your story and then goes to the medicine cabinet for drugs that he or she claims are specific for what ails you. Which of these is a quack, and which one believes in the treatment he or she espouses? I can't read their minds, but I do have a pretty good sense of which treatments are no better than the mustard plaster your grandmother applied to your chest when you had bronchitis. There's nothing wrong with being a true believer, but if you sell the stuff you believe in, you should be able to show evidence that indicates you're right.

I don't mean to point fingers only at people who make and distribute diet supplements and other products. Completely mainstream medical disciplines sometimes have trouble explaining what works and why. Back when I was trying to choose a medical specialty in the 1960s, I remember wondering about psychotherapy as a treatment. There were many different "schools" of psychotherapy, each applying its own principles to understand and change human behavior: the Freudians, the Jungians, the Adlerians, and many more. Members of each group adamantly defended their approaches and argued that their treatments must be working because their patients kept coming back for more sessions. It was not until the late 1970s that studies found that the particular school or philosophy was nowhere near as important as the relation between therapist and patient. As I said before, a good doctor-patient relation is a powerful tool for wellness. Those earlier therapists turned out to be right: when patients returned, it was a pretty good indication that they'd found a given doctor's treatment beneficial—one kind of successful outcome. But what schools those therapists had come from didn't matter a whit.

Some common medical treatments are actually supported by only thin logic—for example, taking thyroid pills when there is no evidence of reduced thyroid function. Here's the logic some doctors (and patients) use. The patient complains of body temperature that is lower than it used to be. The doctor knows that a poorly functioning thyroid gland can lead to low body temperatures, and concludes that the patient must have something wrong with the thyroid. The logic flaw here has to do with what you remember your temperature to have been in the past. Were you aware that average temperature over a twenty-four-hour period is 98.2 degrees and not 98.6 degrees, as we once thought? It turns out that it's normal for your temperature to be lower than 98 degrees at certain times of the day, and body temperature in chronic fatigue syndrome (CFS) patients is no different from that of healthy people. We might know this if we were used to taking our temperature all the time, but of course we don't; we take our temperature only when we feel sick. If you found a temperature of 97.5 degrees in your current health state, it may have startled you, but it is not abnormal. So going on thyroid replacement medicine based on this single reason makes no sense and carries with it unnecessary risks.

## Intravenous Treatments

Some of my CFS patients arrive in my office telling me that they felt better after they've had an intravenous vitamin treatment. With an intravenous drip, a plastic tube is run into your vein, and liquid drips directly into your bloodstream. These intravenous drips are comprised of two elements: a hefty amount of saline (basically saltwater) plus the addition of vitamins and minerals. Dr. David Bell, a pediatrician in New York State, sees many CFS patients. He has given intravenous saline to patients with postural orthostatic tachycardia syndrome (POTS) and reports that they feel substantially better after the volume load. This probably happens because the saline counteracts an overall reduction in blood volume in patients; essentially, they feel better because their veins and arteries are carrying the amount of fluid they were designed to carry (I will discuss this and other research on POTS in the next chapter). But Dr. Bell shares my view that saline alone might do as much as saline loaded with vitamins and minerals. It certainly would be a lot cheaper. But like the psychotherapists in the 1960s, the doctor who chooses infusion therapy is never willing to devote the time or resources to find out if his treatment actually works. And the treatment remains totally unproven. Unfortunately, there is not one bit of evidence that flooding the body with vitamins and minerals has efficacy in any illness or disease. In fact, a carefully done double-blind placebo-controlled study of vitamins and antioxidants taken by mouth proved ineffective at relieving the symptoms of fatigue and soreness in CFS patients.

Some doctors add chemicals to the mix. In a treatment called *chelation therapy*, the practitioner employs a chemical that's normally used to bind heavy metals (like mercury and lead) to treat people poisoned by these metals. Some doctors have the idea that unexplained fatigue and chemical sensitivity are due to heavy metal toxicity. While exposure to heavy metals can cause many symptoms, there is no good evidence that heavy metals have any role at all in CFS, fibromyalgia (FM), multiple chemical sensitivity (MCS), or irritable bowel syndrome (IBS). Despite this, some practitioners frighten patients by telling them the mercury in their dental fillings may be the factor making them sick. This issue has been examined, and there is no evidence to support the assertion. Nonetheless, I have several patients who were convinced of this and went through the long, expensive, and painful process of having all their amalgams removed. Unfortunately, they are still ill. Any believer can act as an authority and state that heavy metals or mercury from teeth are responsible for your being sick. And if there is M.D. or D.O. (Doctor of Osteopathic Medicine) after his or her name, that practitioner can use intravenous chelation as a treatment.

Using chelation as a treatment for CFS or FM is extreme even for believers in chelation. Its major suggested use in alternative medicine is as a treatment to clean out plugged arteries. A number of small controlled studies found no support for this hypothesis, but in 2002, the National Center for Complementary and Alternative Medicine (NCCAM) and the National Heart, Lung, and Blood Institute (NHLBI)—both of are part of the National Institutes of Health—announced that they had launched the Trial to Assess Chelation Therapy. This carefully designed double-blind placebo-controlled trial will tell us about the treatment's efficacy as well as its toxicities. We will have a better idea of whether it works when the trial is completed, but until then I would stay away from this treatment. Even if chelation helps your coronary arteries, that doesn't mean it will do anything for your fatigue.

In fact, I would urge you to be leery of taking any intravenous treatment that hasn't been proven effective. By definition, these treatments introduce drugs and other substances directly into the bloodstream. If any of the materials in the infusion have the potential to be toxic, putting them directly into the bloodstream increases those chances. There's often more than one way to administer a drug; even if it *could* cure the common cold, I doubt you'd want to inject yourself with chicken soup.

## NCCAM and Clinical Research

More research is seldom a bad idea, which is why I'm happy that our government is using taxpayer money to fund NCCAM, whose mission is to support research on using alternative and complementary approaches to develop new treatments for disease. The institute was headed until recently by a smart clinical researcher who was heavily involved in CFS research prior to taking charge of this new institute. His leadership and strong scientific background in experimental design laid the groundwork for the kind of research necessary to discover and test wholly new approaches to treating the invisible illnesses.

Clinical trials have two possible outcomes. The first supports use of the product, device, or treatment for a specific illness. The second does not support that use. A negative result can actually be helpful, because it will usually discourage people from spending limited resources on a treatment with no apparent value. As I was writing this chapter, newspapers were reporting negative results from a large trial of the nutraceutical echinacea for the prevention or treatment of the common cold. I'll give you another example that pertains to fatigue in the next section of this chapter.

The problem with any negative study, on the other hand, is that it cannot *absolutely* prove the negative. One can always say that if the study had been done differently, a different (and more positive) outcome might have occurred. And as I said earlier of our own modafinil study, some individual patients may still be helped even when a well-designed study has negative results. But not all studies are alike. The echinacea study, which was reported in a major American medical journal, the *New England Journal of Medicine*, was particularly thorough. People may continue buying echinacea, but, if it works, it does so because of their belief in its efficacy rather than because it has a specific antiviral effect.

## Nutraceuticals

Echinacea is an example of a nutraceutical, a class of food-based chemicals that are thought to have an effect on health. The number of these products multiplied greatly after Congress passed the Dietary Supplement Health and Education Act (DSHEA), a law that allows the sale of "natural" health products or nutraceuticals with only minimal government oversight. While DSHEA did legislate FDA oversight of these products, the rules governing their use are extremely liberal. Since evidence of effectiveness is not required, the only rule is that nutraceutical manufacturers can't make health claims about their products. So marketers have to be careful not to say that their product can relieve symptoms such as fatigue or pain. Doing so without evidence and FDA approval is illegal, although a glance at just about any health magazine shows ads that do make substantial health claims.

In addition, the entrepreneur selling these products does not have to demonstrate that they are safe. The bottom line is that what is available for purchase—even if "organic"—is not necessarily safe. In fact, I know of one proposed clinical trial at my institution with a nutraceutical that was found to be contaminated with lead. Perhaps just as troubling, nutraceutical manufacturers don't need to set uniform dosages either. Assuming they're even made the same way, two similarly labeled products from different manufacturers might be totally unalike. It's like comparing apples and oranges.

It's important to talk about these products in the context of chronic fatigue and pain, since the long and sometimes difficult course of treatment suggested by classical medicine—or even by valuable complementary therapies—often results in people being tempted by the lure of relief from products that are sometimes expensive but of unknown and probably limited efficacy. Let's look at a few of the dozens of products that are relevant here. I'll start with a few whose effect has been studied.

## Siberian Ginseng

The first is Siberian ginseng for people with CFS. The reason for trying ginseng is that it is thought to be a tonic and stimulant. The ginseng trial was double-blinded. Half the patients received ginseng and the other half placebo. Both groups showed an improvement in their fatigue over the two months of the trial, but the improvement was the same for the two groups. A subgroup analysis suggested that the ginseng treatment did help those patients with less severe fatigue, but there is a problem with subgroup analyses: they tend to be done only when the primary outcome turns out to be negative. When that happens, investigators start sifting through their data in the hopes of finding something useful. And when they try every type of comparison they can think of, they often find a positive result. Statisticians have taught us that this is likely just due to chance and probably would not stand up if the trial were repeated.

Although the law does not require nutraceutical manufacturers to provide proof that their product has a beneficial outcome for any health issue, some companies are willing to support research to see if actual data are as positive as the testimonials they receive about their product. While this is obviously not terribly common, it does occur, and the results that emerge from such studies are worth taking a look at.

## Ambrotose

In addition to the Enerdyn trial I mentioned in the last chapter, I have done another double-blind placebo-controlled trial of a nutraceutical called Ambrotose. Ambrotose is an extract of the aloe plant. The company making this product was willing to pay for the costs of doing the trial due to multiple testimonials about how well their product relieved fatigue and pain. While I think that decision was the right one, our study was negative: we found no evidence that it worked any better than placebo in relieving symptoms of fatigue, poor sleep, and widespread pain.

## BioBran

A rather different example has to do with the nutraceutical Bio-Bran, a product made by breaking down rice bran with enzymes from the shiitake mushroom. In contrast to some heavily promoted nutraceuticals, this food supplement actually seems to do what it is said to do—that is, improve an aspect of immune function. The company selling this food supplement lists dozens of scientific studies, including ones on people, indicating that the product can improve natural killer (NK) cell activity. This is particularly interesting in CFS because immune activation is one of the mechanisms forwarded by some to explain the sick feeling, fatigue, and soreness characteristic of CFS. I'll go into this hypothesis in more detail in the next chapter but need to touch upon NK cell function here. NK cells work to target and kill virally infected cells and tumor cells, so these cells are an important bodily defense against virus infection. Therefore, high numbers of these cells and the ability to easily kill target cells are desirable. Importantly, the one immune variable that has been rather consistently reported to be abnormal in CFS is the NK cell. Some papers report that the numbers of these cells circulating in the blood is reduced, and others say they function less well than they should. Having a product that actually improves the ability of NK cells to kill virally infected cells therefore allows us to see if the NK cell plays an important role in producing CFS.

A double-blind placebo-controlled trial of BioBran over an eight-week period was done with thirty-two CFS patients getting placebo and thirty-two the food supplement. In addition to fulfilling the case definition for CFS, all of the study participants had to have at least two of the following symptoms suggestive of immune activation: tender glands, a sore throat, or something called poor temperature control. The results of the trial were clear. Although both groups improved as to symptom severity over the course of the study, those getting BioBran did not do better than those getting the placebo. The only limitation of this study was that the researchers did not assess NK cell function directly. It is possible that the patients in this study did not have low NK cell numbers or activity to start with and that the study would have been positive if just that group had been identified and randomized. But the researchers did pick patients whose symptoms suggested immune activation. Although BioBran may have worked on other CFS patients, with the group chosen for study, BioBran did not reduce CFS symptoms. A critical take-home message for you is the importance of having the placebo group. Without it, you and others might run to the store to buy BioBran. The other important conclusion from the study is that altered NK cell activity doesn't seem to be an important factor in producing CFS symptoms. Keep this study in mind when I turn to the next nutraceutical, Fibronol.

## Fibronol

I saw a press release saying that the company manufacturing Fibronol had done a clinical trial of their product in FM with striking improvement in energy and moderately large reductions in pain and fatigue. Intrigued, I went to the company Web site and found what seemed like more good news: the trial had apparently been double-blind and placebo-controlled. As in the case of the BioBran study, this should mean that approximately equal numbers of patients got active product and placebo and that neither the patients nor the people administering the trial knew what was being dispensed.

Then I read the following pieces of information. The design called for three groups of ten patients, in which *eight* of the patients received active product and only *two* received the placebo. This occurred for two weeks, and then even the placebo patients were switched to the active product. That certainly did not sound as if "double-blind placebo-controlled" to me. Instead, it sounded as if the vast majority of patients received only Fibronol, and the few who started out on the placebo were switched to Fibronol shortly after starting the trial as well.

Then the information got even more confusing. Somehow, the study was conducted in ten "centers," with twenty-two patients in Korea and fourteen in Seattle. How ten centers in two countries recruited thirty-six patients is beyond me. If true, this means that ten different doctors ran the trial, and each center had an average of only four patients—very unusual indeed. Usually treatment trials seek to recruit substantially more patients from each site. And it got still more complicated. Some of the patients, it turns out, were put on a high dose and some on a lower dose of Fibronol. By now, you should be as confused as I was.

Then I turned to the objectives of the study. One was to demonstrate the safety of Fibronol. Secondary aims were to see if a single dose of Fibronol improved pain or fatigue and to see if high dose was better than a lower dose. What was absent? The key objective: to see whether Fibronol worked or not compared to placebo.

As to the primary objective, Fibronol seemed relatively safe, although 20 percent of the patients could not tolerate taking this product and dropped out during the study—most for worsening problems with preexisting diarrhea. I couldn't find any information on outcomes concerning the secondary aims of the study, but there was plenty of attention to symptom improvement, even though there didn't seem to be any comparisons between product and placebo. Why did the patients improve on Fibronol? Due to the design of the study, we can't know if symptom improvement was due to the nutraceutical or to the placebo effect. Using the BioBran trial as a point of reference, this study was of such poor quality that it would never be published in the medical literature.

Thus the company simply bypassed that process and put the study on the Internet.

## Buyer Beware

I ask myself how such companies manage to be so successful. And successful they are. The company selling Ambrotose reported selling $194 million worth of products in 2004. One obvious answer is that these companies do not publish negative data, like those in my Ambrotose trial. Or they pick the results that make the best case for their product even if the findings were not part of the original study design, as seems to have been the case with Fibronol. This careful editing out of negative results, and massaging of the rest, of course multiplies the hope that these products engender. Add to that the desperation of so many patients to believe in self-proclaimed "cures," and it's much easier to see why they sell.

But there is another factor. These companies take a leaf from the old "Avon calling" salesbook, using multilevel marketing. In this method, an individual patient can greatly reduce the cost of buying product—and actually earn a living—by using the product and extolling its value to others. A one-month supply of Fibronol costs about $79, which is comparable to the cost of many of the drugs I recommended in chapter 7 (except that those are often covered by insurance). Buying the product in quantity does reduce the cost, but you still have to lay out a lot of money. If you can get a few friends or fellow patients to sell the product, however, your cost goes down considerably. And if they can get a few of their friends to successfully sell the product, you can be in business and actually start making money. Imagine how this situation might magnify a placebo effect. You're sick and someone tells you they felt energized when they took this food supplement. They tell you to try it, then if you like it, you can get it less expensively if you become a seller yourself. Moreover, you can make money selling the product to other patients. That's powerful medicine!

The bottom line, of course, must always be improved health—wellness. But you should remain aware that many companies peddling health nutritional supplements may be selling a very expensive form of hope. Only real, controlled research will show which of these products, if any, have a demonstrable effect on CFS, FM, and the other unexplained illnesses. The BioBran story makes the point that some of these food supplements can alter biological processes that have an impact on health. But the company making this product paid for quite a large number of studies documenting the immune-activating power of their product. Look for lists of such evidence when you evaluate the Web site of a company selling a nutraceutical for CFS, FM, temporomandibular joint disorder (TMD), and the like. Be sure that the list includes reports in scientific journals and not just reports at medical meetings. These latter have not received the careful, independent scrutiny of papers published in the scientific or medical literature. If the company Web site lists no studies or only a few reports at medical or scientific meetings, be skeptical about the company's claims. Without saying these products are absolutely bogus, I can at least point to the historical track record. Nutritional supplements of one kind or another have always existed, and we've all heard about cure-alls of the past that were later debunked. The old rule of buyer beware is even more important when your health hangs in the balance.

In addition to companies selling hope, there are doctors who do the same thing. They make promises of wellness tied to easy (and/or expensive) cures. If the solution to your illness were "easy," you would not be sick now. But there is a way to cope with illness—the path to wellness that I laid out in part 2 of this book. It is not easy, and does demand your active participation. But if you commit to it, you will feel better. I too am selling hope: the hope that you can improve your own health without paying thousands of dollars to do so.

# 11

# Promising Research into the "Invisible Illnesses"

Besides wanting to know how I can help them right away, most of my patients want to know the latest news about their illnesses, and whether new treatments are on the horizon. Ironically, invisible illnesses are one area where patients are often more up to date than their physicians. But since my patients know that one of my major focus areas is research, they expect to hear from me things that they can't find out for themselves.

My patients are right about my focus on research. But it's also true that medical knowledge grows very slowly; sometimes it feels as if the gods are against us researchers. If anything can go wrong in a research project, it certainly will, at least for a time. And the actual work of doing laboratory and clinical research is incredibly slow even when everything is working beautifully.

So when I tell interested patients that there is not much new since the last visit, I can understand the disappointment. However, that's the way research goes—by microsteps, until all of a sudden the little bits of information add up to allow the researcher to make a discernible step forward. These statements are true of research in general, but even more so for illnesses with no biomarkers. I liken my own research to sculpting granite with a rubber chisel—apt to bear results, but not very quickly.

You might wonder why I am so committed to research. Because

when I knock a chip off that granite block, and it starts to take a form, I am the first person to see the truth. That is the thrill of discovery, the joy of understanding just a little bit more than we did before. Being the first person to see and understand a biological or medical truth is a wonderful experience, and an ample reward for hours and sometimes years of hard work.

## The Idea of Truth or Fact in Science

In this chapter, I'm going to describe the latest advances that research has brought us in understanding syndromic illness, but first it's important to discuss the basic idea of facts in research. The bottom line is that what scientists *know* to be true today may not be true tomorrow. New knowledge sometimes proves that what was thought to be a fact is not. This is partly because science plants one fact on top of a foundation of earlier facts and these new facts can actually modify the old ones. But science is also built on the repetition of experiments by other researchers, to confirm that the original research reached the right conclusions for the right reasons. Sometimes, these repeat experiments lead instead to different and unexpected outcomes. So over time, our understanding about any area in science or medicine slowly changes. The principal driver of this change is the researcher's need to replicate a finding.

Chronic mononucleosis is one case where research changed doctors' understanding of the facts. Acute infectious mononucleosis starts quite suddenly with symptoms of severe fatigue and a sore throat; on examination, the patient will usually show a fever, a red throat, and swollen glands in the neck and armpits. You will recall that mono is caused by infection with several viruses in the *herpesvirus* family, most commonly the Epstein-Barr virus (EBV). For many years, when a person came down with mono but never recovered fully, it seemed likely that the patient had chronic mononucleosis. In the 1980s, this became an accepted diagnosis, and it seemed reasonable since these people appeared to have evidence of chronically active EBV infection: elevated antibodies to the virus. So the idea that there was a chronic form of mononucleosis became a fact, and doctors began ordering EBV tests for patients whose fatigue had no apparent medical cause.

Here's the problem: subsequent work showed that almost *everyone* had elevated levels of these antibodies, because most of us are exposed to EBV as kids (it usually takes the form of just another sore throat). So much for chronic mono, which was subsequently renamed chronic fatigue syndrome (CFS). The symptoms were real enough, but the explanation that had seemed like a fact no longer made sense. While other studies have found that these patients tend to have higher EBV antibody levels than healthy people, there is an enormous overlap. Today, we know that there are no convincing data showing that persisting viral infection is the cause of illnesses like CFS. However, the chronic viral infection hypothesis persists for other viruses. I will discuss those possibilities later in this chapter.

## How Research Answers Questions

There are a number of different approaches to understanding the causes of a clinical illness. These approaches are quite different from those we use when we're trying to understand basic biological questions, such as how a cell works. That's called basic research. Clinical research may be very hands-on, with patients actively involved in experiments, or it may be applied, with a researcher comparing biological samples from patients—for example, blood or muscle tissue—to those from healthy comparison subjects. In this way, scientists can discover differences that might lead to an understanding of the biology of the disease.

Another kind of clinical research consists of doing drug trials. Drug trials have two purposes: to develop new treatments to help patients with a disease, and to prove specific ideas about how a given disease is caused. I gave you one example in the last chapter when I discussed the BioBran trial. A positive outcome would have provided ammunition for the immune dysfunction hypothesis as the cause of CFS. Another example was a trial of an antiviral medication in people with CFS. If the patients improved, that result would have supported the idea that an active viral infection, such as chronic mononucleosis, was responsible for CFS. However, that was not the outcome. The people receiving the treatment—one to eradicate EBV—showed no more improvement than those receiving a placebo.

My patients know that I am a researcher, so they often wonder whether I'm wearing my doctor hat or my researcher hat when I recommend a given course of treatment. I can understand this confusion because I ask some of my patients to participate in my research. It's easy to tell the difference between doctorly advice and actual research, however, since no one can be part of a study without signing a form known as a research informed consent. This document explains exactly what participating in a study will involve, and any risks that may arise. Nowadays, research cannot be done without your informed consent. If you do not have a document indicating that you have given your consent to participate in research, no one is allowed to conduct research in which you're a subject. But it's wonderful when people take the opportunity to participate in research, because this is how medical advances are really made. If the afflicted did not volunteer to participate in research on the invisible illnesses, we'd never be able to move ahead.

Now that you have a sense of what research is about and the importance of participating in it, I'll describe the most cutting-edge research areas and why some of them are so promising and exciting. I've worked to make these understandable because I've found that my patients are always curious about, and fascinated by, the latest research directions. Based on past experience with my patients, I'm sure you'll be able to digest the science that follows.

## Genetic Research

As in many areas of medicine, some of the key research into medically unexplained illnesses today involves inheritance, or genetics. The most powerful way to study inheritance is to examine pairs of twins, in which one twin is healthy while the other exhibits a medical problem. If the problem relates to inheritance, then the rates of disease will be higher in identical twin pairs than in nonidentical twin pairs. If the problem relates to situations within the environment, then the rates of disease should be equal in identical and nonidentical twins—that is, assuming they don't live in radically different environments. Two groups have conducted research into chronic fatigue with twins as the subjects, and both reported similar results—the rates of fatigue were higher in a group of sick identical twins than in a group of sick nonidentical twins. That was an important finding, especially coming from two different studies, because it showed that a tendency toward chronic fatigue could be inherited; in other words, it may run in your family.

One of the studies found an equally important second result: that fatigue and depression did not go hand in hand but instead had independent risks related to inheritance. Another group used a second approach—the family method—to look at the question of heredity in fibromyalgia (FM). In the family method, researchers ask questions over the phone to ascertain if a relative of the patient has the same medical condition or symptom, in this case, medically unexplained pain. The researchers found that FM existed in 19 percent of the relatives of patients with FM but in only 4 percent of the relatives of patients with rheumatoid arthritis (RA). The group also found a raised rate of depression in the relatives of FM patients compared to what was found in relatives of RA patients. The fact that this association was not found in chronic fatigue suggests that illnesses characterized primarily by fatigue may differ from illnesses characterized primarily by pain. Depression and pain may be linked somehow, while depression and fatigue are not. But finding a link between FM and depression is important in and of itself. The results of the studies just mentioned suggest that whatever produces FM also may produce depression, a possibility I discussed in chapter 5.

One major problem with this family method study is that the researchers did not confirm the diagnosis of FM by doing a tender point exam. To remind you, the diagnosis of FM requires widespread pain plus multiple tender points. However, in the family study performed by my colleague Dr. Karen Raphael, she rectified this problem by assessing people for tender points too. She found the same result: family members of patients with FM had an increased risk for having both FM and depression and not necessarily at the same time. As in the family study conducted without a tender point exam, the increased risk was about 20 percent. Obviously this is a lot less than half, so we can deduce that genetics are not the whole explanation. But the studies do add up to mean that inheritance is one factor in producing medically unexplained fatigue and pain. Such a link is important because it indicates that these illnesses should not be in the "nothing wrong" category; they exist and have a genetic explanation, at least for some patients.

Finally, a group at the University of North Carolina has made a major step ahead in understanding how genetic predisposition can lead to pain-related problems. This group genotyped 202 healthy women, looking specifically for different forms of a gene related to pain sensitivity called COMT; prior to this work, interest in this gene was mostly focused on the fact that its primary action was to produce the hormone adrenaline. Importantly, the researchers found that specific forms of the gene predicted increased sensitivity to painful stimuli. Over the three years of the study, fifteen women developed temporomandibular joint disorder (TMD); of these, half had the genotype for increased pain. Yes, this is a small number, but the results will encourage further research—again with the goal of replicating this result. Nonetheless, this result suggests that genetic factors play an important role in the development of this regional pain syndrome. My guess is that the same genetic sensitivity will be shown to be important in irritable bowel syndrome (IBS) as well as in FM. Being able to pinpoint a gene is the first step in coming up with therapies to reduce its role in magnifying the intensity of a painful stimulus.

## The Immune System Connection

Some of my own research has looked at the idea that the immune system may be involved in chronic fatigue and pain. In the same way that early work suggested that viral infection might be the cause of isolated fatigue and widespread pain, similar logic implicated the immune system. When you get the flu, it is not the virus that makes you feel awful; instead, it is your body's *response* to the virus that causes symptoms like elevated temperature and fatigue. Unpleasant though the result may be—no one likes to be bedridden with the flu—we can take some small comfort from knowing that if we feel awful, our body is probably trying to fight the infection. Researchers reasoned that in the case of many diseases, it is the factors that produce the immune response that protect a person from infection.

Over the past decade, drug companies have worked hard to isolate these immune active materials, which are called *cytokines*. In studying the actions of cytokines, researchers learned that they can also improve health in diseases with dysregulated cytokine release or viral infection. Therefore the pharmaceutical industry has invested many millions of dollars to develop cytokines—or substances that neutralize the actions of cytokines—for use as drugs. Currently, cytokines or cytokine blockers are used in the treatment of autoimmune and virally related diseases including multiple sclerosis, rheumatoid arthritis, and hepatitis. And researchers are working hard to identify other diseases that could be improved by manipulating immune activity.

When cytokines are given to a person, the drug itself makes the person sick—just as in the case when the body makes cytokines as a reaction to viral infection. Realizing that cytokines given as drugs often produced flulike symptoms and diffuse soreness, researchers began to hypothesize that unexplained pain and fatigue had an immunological basis. In fact, patient advocates initially labeled patients with prolonged and disabling fatigue as having chronic fatigue and immune dysfunction syndrome (CFIDS).

This idea led to a flurry of research in the 1980s and early 1990s that found immunological abnormalities in people with CFS, which also extended to people with other unexplained illnesses, such as FM. Focus on CFS was most intense because of the flulike symptoms that were part and parcel of that illness. However, research done to try to replicate these early reports, including our own, found relatively little difference in the immune function of patients and of healthy people.

One explanation for this result lay in the fact that data from extremely sedentary patients were compared to data from active healthy people; these differences in activity or fitness alone can explain much of the difference between patients and controls. However, our own careful review of the immunological literature noted that one test—for natural killer (NK) cells—was frequently abnormal across studies, with either low numbers of cells in the blood or low activity of existing cells. High counts and high activity are thought to be healthful in that the job of these cells is to target and kill virally infected cells and tumor cells.

Importantly, new evidence exists to indicate that these results are not simply due to differences in activity between the healthy comparison group and the patients. A recent study from the University of Miami found the same reductions in patients compared to sedentary but otherwise well controls. In addition, they found that those patients with low NK cell activity have more symptoms and do worse on cognitive tests than those with normal levels. Finding objective differences in cognitive function is important and does suggest using NK cells as a marker of a subgroup of patients with immune dysfunction. However, as I discussed in the last chapter, BioBran, a nutraceutical that increases NK cell activity, did not improve CFS symptoms. This negative result leads me to conclude that NK cell dysfunction is not a cause of the disease but a marker perhaps related to disease severity or inactivity. But identifying markers is still very important in allowing us to identify subgroups of patients that each may have different reasons for illness onset.

Besides the NK story, there really is little to support the idea of immune dysfunction as a cause of medically unexplained fatigue and achiness. But here's an interesting twist: Digging a little deeper into the research, I learned that all of the studies looking for all types of immune differences had looked at blood drawn during the daytime. What happens at night might also be well worth studying and nocturnal alterations in immune function might produce chronic fatigue and pain by disturbing sleep.

The immune system is known to regulate sleep via a balance between sleep-producing and sleep-disturbing cytokines. Perhaps some patients had a disease of cytokine regulation in which the normal balance of the different kinds of cytokines was tilted in favor of sleep-disturbing cytokines, resulting in night after night of poor sleep. Obviously such people would have fatigue, and some data existed to indicate that they would have pain too. In contrast to this, I thought that poor sleepers—people with insomnia—would show an imbalance in favor of sleep-producing cytokines.

As we discussed in chapter 6, unrefreshing sleep is a hallmark of medically unexplained fatigue and pain, and sleep studies in patients with these problems found disrupted sleep with frequent periods of awakening throughout the night. My idea was to sample sleep-producing and sleep-disturbing cytokines while CFS patients and healthy comparison subjects slept. If my hypothesis of a disturbed cytokine sleep network in patients with FM and CFS was correct, then a night of total sleep deprivation for both patients and healthy controls should magnify the differences. The sleep cytokine network of healthy people should tilt toward sleep-producing cytokines to compensate for the abnormal situation, leading them to fall asleep quickly. But the unhealthy patients, unable to produce sleep-producing cytokines in sufficient numbers (or with sufficient function), probably wouldn't be able to get to sleep despite their fatigue, because of their underlying immune dysfunction. Instead—if I were right—they would still overproduce the sleep-disturbing cytokines and continue to show problems falling asleep.

My proposal to study the sleep-cytokine system in CFS was finally approved by the National Institutes of Health (NIH). As I write this chapter, the work has been going on for more than two years. Women with CFS are coming to our university for medical evaluation and, when appropriate for research, they return to our laboratory for blood sampling while they sleep. If you're curious about how the work is going, I'm afraid you'll have to be patient a while longer; but in 2008, you should be able to find the results in medical journals. Just type "PubMed" into any Web search engine and then enter my name, and you'll be able to find the National Library of Medicine's list of articles.

So, if I am right, I will have found an explanation for some cases of what had been labeled as "medically unexplained illness"—an immune dysfunction that robs some patients of adequate rest. As I explained in the early chapters of this book, this incremental approach is the way medicine advances. But even if my hypothesis is correct, I have to emphasize that it really will apply only to some cases. I don't expect it to hold for those patients who complain of unrefreshing sleep but who actually have normal sleep patterns. In contrast, my hypothesis should hold for those patients whose sleep is shown to be characterized by multiple mini-arousals—brief episodes of wakefulness of which they might not even be aware. And then what? I will work with pharmaceutical companies to develop a drug to right the imbalance, either by blocking the action of the sleep-disturbing cytokines or by increasing the release of the sleep-producing cytokines. But, obviously, all this will take time.

I also gave some thought to the fact that nearly every study on immune function had looked within blood. That left out a whole range of other possibilities. One of the first studies I ever did showed that patients with fatiguing illness—produced by CFS or MS—also had cognitive problems. As a neurologist, I immediately came up with the idea that some patients with fatigue might actually experience their symptoms due to a brain problem. It occurred to me that the place to look for immune abnormalities might be the fluid that bathes the brain—spinal fluid—rather than blood. To evaluate that idea, I conducted a study in which I collected spinal fluid from patients with CFS, as well as from healthy comparison subjects.

The spinal tap—also known as a lumbar puncture—sounds scary to many people, but research has shown that most people find it less uncomfortable than getting an injection in the buttocks. And in this case, the discomfort may well have been worth it, because our study found two potentially important results: first, 30 percent of the patients had minor abnormalities in the makeup of their spinal fluid, but *none* of the people in the healthy control group showed these abnormalities. Second, I found increases in one cytokine for CFS patients with sudden illness onset, and increases in a different cytokine for those who had the abnormal spinal fluid results. These results certainly should put to rest the idea that patients with this disorder have the "nothing wrong syndrome." This study is particularly important because it is one of the first to document immune dysfunction related to the brain.

## The Role of the Brain and the Heart

These results with cytokines supported our earlier work suggesting that some people with CFS have a subtle neurological disorder. In those earlier studies, we had found that CFS patients with no evidence of depression were the ones with *worse* cognitive function than CFS patients who had experienced depression. The way we check cognitive function is to conduct neuropsychological tests. The complaint of fuzzy brain, while fairly common in CFS patients, usually expresses itself only in subtle ways, but neuropsych testing showed problems in doing at least one set of tasks: those that require both mental processing and a physical, motor response. (As an example of this, we might ask a patient to look at a series of numbers on a computer—the processing part of the test—and press a button to indicate whether the newest number is the same as the one that appeared two numbers before (the "motor" part).

A second important finding was that people who had never been depressed had more abnormalities on brain magnetic resonance imaging (MRI tests) than people who had also suffered with depression. These abnormalities were usually tiny lesions, few in number, and they could occur in healthy people too—but only rarely. Some evidence exists suggesting that these MRI abnormalities are only the tip of an iceberg. A recent report indicated that the part of the brain responsible for cognitive processing, called the cerebral cortex, was smaller in CFS patients without evidence of depression than in healthy people. Patients who were the least active had smaller cerebral cortical volumes than those who were more active. Although it is possible that this was a product of inactivity, the more likely explanation is that the results reflect some smoldering ongoing disease process.

The bottom line is that some form of brain dysfunction, which can be measured and which may take a physical form, may be the cause of your severe fatigue and pain. To a neurologist, the combination of mild cognitive problems, minor abnormalities on brain magnetic resonance imaging, and minor abnormalities in spinal fluid—in the absence of depression—adds up to something wrong with the brain, but just how they do so is a question for further research. No one wants to have brain dysfunction, of course, but where there are physical abnormalities, there is always a hope of treatment. And at the very least, this procession of studies pointing to differences in brain function—or even in the physical condition of the brain—is early evidence of an explanation for illnesses that had previously been thought to have no medical explanation, or even worse, were imaginary.

To shed more light on how we carried out all this research, it's worth talking about how MRI scans work. You've probably heard of these tests, which enable doctors to see the anatomy of everything under the skin, but few people are really aware of how they work. The most common application of MRI is to look for anatomical abnormalities. The scans work by imaging the amount of water in different bodily tissues, with bone having the least and spinal fluid or blood having the most. The slight differences in water composition within the brain, for example, lets doctors easily differentiate the part of the brain housing the brain cells, called neurons, from the neighboring fiber tracks connecting those neurons with one another. And seeing a tumor or an abnormal collection of blood vessels is easy with MRI. In contrast, functional magnetic resonance imaging moves past anatomy; it can localize the part of the brain responsible for different bodily functions or different feeling states.

As an example, let's consider how an MRI would show the part of the brain that's active when I tap my finger on a desk. In order to tap my finger, the neurons that control the muscles in my finger need to turn on. Active cells require oxygen and the body's major nutrient, glucose, in order to continue working efficiently. To get these substances to the brain cells that are suddenly active when I wish to tap my finger, blood vessels near those cells open up (dilate), bringing more oxygen into the working cells. The detectors in the MRI scanner can sense the change in oxygen, and so when the brain is imaged, the area housing the active cells lights up.

My colleagues used functional neuroimaging during a mentally challenging task given to CFS patients and during the time that a warm, nonpainful stimulus was applied to the hands of FM patients. Despite very different stimuli and different patient groups, the general outcomes were surprisingly similar. The brains of the CFS patients acted as if the task was much harder than it actually was, while the brains of the FM patients acted as if the stimulus was painfully hot rather than warm. In other words, a healthy person would have to have been given a very difficult task, or subjected to a much more painful stimulus, to produce the same response that the CFS and FM patients experienced when receiving rather easy tasks and stimuli that weren't painful at all. Why the brain overreacts to these inputs is not known, but FM researchers speculate that muscle injury may alter inputs to the brain in such a way to lead to this kind of sensitized response.

While these results could suggest that the brains of all the patients were set at a higher notch than would be the case for healthy people, another explanation could be that the CFS and FM patients were hyperalert to any stimuli—more expectant that something was going to happen. However, if that were the case, one would expect to see areas of the brain involved in arousal or anticipation to light up also, and this was not the case. So the idea of hyperalertness does not really explain a major finding in fibromyalgia—that FM patients report pain when they're subjected to lower amounts of physical pressure than people without this problem. That this was not the case suggests that painful (or even not-so-painful) stimuli cause the brains of these patients to overreact; this is called central sensitization. That interpretation is buttressed by experiments showing that FM patients show a distinctly different physiological response to a painful stimulus from healthy controls. People with both FM and IBS show the same reduction in pain threshold as patients with FM alone. Oddly enough, though, when IBS occurs without FM, the situation changes; these patients are actually less sensitive to pain in most parts of the body, but they're hypersensitive to the painful stimulus of rectal distention. This result may mean that IBS alone is a different disease from IBS with FM.

A rather different way of looking for brain dysfunction is to see how the brain responds when it is activated. A common way to do this in the laboratory is to impose a stressful demand—a physical stress like vigorous exercise, or a mental stress like asking the subject to do math computations in his or her head. Researchers then gauge brain activation by looking at the organs the brain controls, such as the heart, the blood vessels, and the gut. These organs receive their instructions from the brain via the autonomic nervous system (ANS), and the brain can alter the function of these organs by turning the ANS on or off. The ANS has two branches: the *sympathetic* nervous system that prepares the body for a "fight or flight" reaction, and the *parasympathetic* nervous system that prepares the body for eating, digestion, and sex.

When the body gets ready to run or fight, digestion stops, sexual arousal withers, heart rate and blood pressure zoom, and the adrenal gland pumps out two hormones: adrenalin, which improves alertness and further turns on the cardiovascular system, and a variant of cortisone called cortisol, which works to release the body's major fuel, glucose, from its storage reservoir in the liver. Now the body has plenty of fuel, enabling you to run, fight, or do whatever else you need to do to protect yourself from imminent danger. Once the emergency is over, everything returns to normal, and the sympathetic and parasympathetic limbs of the ANS come back into balance. In contrast, when you are eating or resting, your parasympathetic nervous system takes the lead.

You now know that when people with unexplained symptoms are stressed, their brains tend to overreact compared to the brains of healthy people in a control group. You would think that the body, responding to this increased brain activity, would also become even more poised for "fight or flight" than the bodies of healthy people. Instead, the opposite happens: in people with CFS and the other "unexplained" illnesses, the body actually responds *less*! So if you have one of these illnesses and you suddenly find yourself in a stressful situation, you'll actually experience a double whammy: Your brain will work harder, but your body will be *less* responsive. Perhaps this combination of mild biological deficiencies adds up to produce the dramatic symptom worsening that people report after even minimal effort.

This line of research has led to the idea that medically unexplained fatigue and pain may be stress-related disorders. A reduced cardiovascular stress response could explain why patients report feeling so much worse after even relatively minor physical or mental stress. The brain is alert, but the heart doesn't pump enough blood to meet the need; when that happens, your organs may not get enough oxygen. You feel stressed, but instead of being poised for action, you feel sluggish.

In addition to reduced "stress reactivity," another measurable difference in people experiencing these illnesses is abnormal day-to-day activity of the stress hormone cortisol, which varies from being on the low side for CFS to being on the high side in TMD. Low levels are associated with fatigue and reduced capacity to deal with infection while high levels over long periods of time can lead to cognitive problems. In addition, there are data—clearer for FM than for CFS or IBS—that stressful life events can trigger the start of these illnesses.

What about the autonomic nervous system, which is supposed to be carrying all of those instructions from your brain to various parts of your body? We know that when healthy people keep physically fit, their ANS balance tilts in favor of increased parasympathetic tone; that's why athletes have such slow heart rates. Deconditioning and disease, on the other hand, reduce paraysmpathetic tone, leading to a predominance of sympathetic tone. Your heart rate increases and you'll feel more stressed.

Our group was one of the first to note that parasympathetic activity was below normal in people with CFS, and the way we did this is interesting. Feel for your pulse, either in your wrist or just to the side of your windpipe in your neck. Breathe in very slowly and then breathe out very slowly. You may feel your pulse rate slow down as you breathe in, and speed up as you breathe out. This "heart rate variability" is due to coupling between breathing and pulse and is called the *respiratory sinus arrhythmia*. It is produced when the parasympathetic nerves connecting your brain to your heart cycle on and off, and is totally normal. Naturally, then, losing this kind of arrhythmia is abnormal. The more clocklike the pulse rate, the poorer the parasympathetic tone. People with diseases such as diabetes, heart failure, CFS, FM, and IBS may find that their pulse does not vary greatly with breathing. This sounds like a good thing, but actually it isn't. Reduced parasympathetic activity means that sympathetic nerves are working more than they should.

To combat this imbalance, I suggested you consider buying Freeze-Framer, the biofeedback software I described in chapter 9. That computer program shows just how well your parasympathetic nerves to the heart are working and allows you to practice improving your parasympathetic tone. Kundalini yoga probably does much the same thing because of its attention to breathing.

Abnormalities in autonomic balance in favor of the sympathetic branch may explain why some CFS patients have a heart rate problem. Remember that when the sympathetic nerves fire, your heart rate goes up. Consistent with their having increased sympathetic tone, some CFS patients have heart rates that are either too high or too reactive. Either their pulse rate at rest is rapid, over 90 beats per minute, or their pulse rate increases by more than 29 beats per minute while standing or hits an absolute value of 120. In the 1980s, when women with these reactive hearts also reported having symptoms of fatigue, chest discomfort, and feeling worse after exertion or after standing, they were usually referred to cardiologists to be sure they didn't have heart disease. Such women received the diagnosis of mitral valve prolapse, a condition where blood sometimes backs up in the heart due to a malfunctioning heart valve. However, advances in cardiac imaging made it clear that these women did not have any heart abnormalities. They were no longer given unnecessary referrals to cardiologists, but unfortunately they were instead left to fend for themselves. They were among the many classes of patients who fell through the cracks of classical medicine.

In the late 1990s, this reactive heart problem was given a new name: postural orthostatic tachycardia syndrome, or POTS. I touched upon this issue in chapter 9. Translated into English, POTS is the syndrome of excessive heart rate acceleration after a person goes from the lying to the standing posture, and it is age-related. POTS is very common in kids with CFS and a lot less common in CFS patients in their late thirties and forties, the average age group of patients in my practice. In contrast, we have recently learned that about 20 percent of our older patients have a different problem related to standing. We call this postural orthostatic syndrome of hyperventilation, or POSH. Here instead of the heart rate zooming, people breathe more deeply and effectively hyperventilate. In doing this, people exhale the carbon dioxide dissolved in their blood more than would normally be the case. Low levels of carbon dioxide in the body produce a host of symptoms, and one early notion—which my colleagues and I examined and rejected years ago—was that CFS was nothing other than hyperventilation syndrome.

In reality, however, hyperventilation and POSH are quite different. A major difference is that CFS patients with POSH breathe normally when lying quietly; it's only when they stand that they change the way they breathe. Nor were our patients hyperventilating (in the usual sense) because they were anxious; our research shows that anxiety and depression scores are the same for CFS patients with POSH as for those without it.

POSH can coexist with POTS. And CFS patients with either POTS, POSH, or both of these abnormal conditions feel worse when they stand than CFS patients without them. Their presence certainly tells us *something*. One similarity between POSH and POTS is that patients with either one have less blood in their chest than is normal. Intrathoracic hypovolemia is normal when you quickly transition from lying to standing. Switching your posture like this leaves a pint of blood—the amount you would donate in a blood drive—behind in the veins of the legs and buttocks, thus temporarily shortchanging the brain. That's why some people get slightly dizzy when they stand up too fast—especially if they've been out in the sun, where the heat causes blood vessels to dilate and pool more blood than when they are constricted (which occurs when you are cold). If you're a healthy person and suddenly stand up on the beach on a hot day, you might experience this dizzy feeling for a moment, only to have it pass quickly. The dizzy feeling has to do with less blood getting to your brain than should be.

Your body is set to deal with these minor orthostatic stresses and does so by adjusting heart rate and blood pressure, so that blood flow to the brain remains normal. But certain patients—very often with complaints of chronic fatigue and achiness—don't show these normal reactions. For reasons researchers are still studying, these patients instead develop POTS, POSH, or both of these physiological abnormalities while stating that they feel a lot worse when they stand up. This symptom is known as orthostatic intolerance, and our working idea is that orthostatic intolerance may lead to reduced blood flow to the brain, which may produce chronic fatigue.

While nothing is known about the physiological processes producing POSH, quite a lot is known about POTS. It seems to develop via several possible mechanisms: because blood exudes out of vessels in the legs into the tissues beneath the skin to produce swelling or edema, because the muscles in the leg that usually pump blood up into the chest don't work well, because blood pools somewhere below the chest, or because there is too little blood altogether. Currently laboratory methods allow us to identify only the last of these. This is done by a radiological test to determine total blood volume and mass of red blood cells. But I have little doubt that research will lead to a better understanding of the rest of these symptoms and of POSH, and that's why these subjects are a cornerstone of my own research goals for the rest of this decade.

Why am I stressing POTS and POSH so much? They fill a gap in trying to understand chronic fatigue. I made a big point earlier in the book about splitting syndromes into subgroups that might allow us to better understand cause and then move on to treatment. My efforts in doing this depended on what patients told me about their illness. In contrast, POTS and POSH produce frank abnormalities that I can measure. They are biological markers for an underlying physiological abnormality that may explain chronic fatigue and widespread pain. Having a physical abnormality provides me more secure ground for splitting patients into groups than would be the case with patient-reported symptoms. Then I can focus on that subgroup in an effort to find its underlying causes and then develop ways of treating or interfering with this process. This process is what is needed to move from the "nothing wrong" explanation to the idea that something definitely is wrong. Diagnosing POTS or POSH in a CFS or FM patient is the way to move ahead with this plan.

What appears to be low blood volume could explain an important finding we have recently made. We divided our CFS patients into those on the severe end of the illness spectrum and those with less-severe CFS. We called a case "severe" if it fulfilled the original 1988 case definition for CFS with symptoms reported to be substantial, severe, or very severe (rather than mild or moderate). We then measured the amount of blood the patients' hearts pumped with each beat (that is, stroke volume). Those with severe CFS had lower stroke volume than less severely ill CFS patients or the healthy controls. If sufficient amounts of blood do not reach the heart—as would be the case with low blood volume—then stroke volume will be low. But stroke volume can also be low if something is wrong with the heart. One of the earliest symptoms of cardiac dysfunction is exertion-related fatigue.

Could underlying heart disease cause CFS? We certainly know that if a heart is damaged either by a heart attack, infection, or having to pump against pressure, as in the case of hypertension, the heart goes through a lengthy process of dealing with the insult. Often, it doesn't completely recover. This is the first step toward heart failure, and it can be decades before the patient has visible signs of this problem, including swollen legs and shortness of breath when lying flat. One group of researchers has suggested that some CFS patients may really have chronic viral infections of the heart. Though they were unable to find an actual virus, they did find antibodies to viral building blocks in some CFS patients. This is an important hypothesis that we are also pursuing, but I don't think it will prove to be a major factor for many CFS patients. In sixteen years of practice, I have not seen one patient go on to develop anything suggestive of heart failure.

The idea that some infectious viral or bacterial agent, or a fragment of such an agent, causes CFS or FM continues despite many negative studies. My own experience with treating possible bacterial infection is equally negative. Since I have never seen a patient improve while on antibiotics, I ask patients to stop taking them if they tell me they are taking them chronically. I believe patients should not receive treatment for infectious agents unless testing definitively confirms infection, because the medicines used to treat infections have marked side effects and can be dangerous. Nonetheless, there is one line of research that supports the idea of chronic infection. Studies that began at Temple University showed that CFS patients have activation of the body's innate antiviral defense mechanisms, a system that normally goes into play only if there's a viral infection. This finding has been replicated in several labs and the system is not activated in fatigue related to depression. Whether this activation reflects a specific underlying infection is not known, but I think research in this direction is important and bears watching in the next few years.

A final possibility is infection of muscle. Early on, some researchers supposed that abnormalities in muscle tissue—infections or some other kind—might explain the muscle achiness of FM and CFS. One recent paper reported finding evidence for viral infection of muscle in 21 percent of CFS patients and in no controls. Those patients positive for infection had more problems on exercise testing than those without infection. This suggests that an infection had affected their ability to use their muscles to exercise. Again, we need to wait for this study to be replicated by others. The research process is a slow one, but I'm confident it will eventually tell us, once and for all, whether some form of infection is responsible for medically unexplained fatigue or pain.

The excitement of research is being able to sort out this tangled web of possibilities. Though we don't yet have final answers for the causes of CFS, FM, and the other illnesses that are the concern of this book, I think some of the most promising research of all is in progress now. And of all of this research, studies on the autonomic nerves, muscles, and vascular control—the bodily systems we've looked at in this chapter—are among the most promising. These studies are likely to find physiological causes for the symptoms of many patients, and perhaps for you.

The very fact that this chapter exists means that despite millions of dollars of research and a great deal of hard work by thousands of scientists, doctors, and patients, we still haven't arrived at a

commonly agreed upon cause of multisymptom illness characterized by fatigue and pain; for the most part, they do remain medically unexplained. Understanding POTS is certainly a step ahead,
and I hope to do the same for POSH in the next few years. It's
heartening to know that the quality of research in understanding
the causes of chronic fatigue and both widespread and localized
pain is improving every year. As a result, we're way beyond where
we were one or two decades ago. I believe that further study of the
heart, blood vessels, brain, and the linkages among them will produce the answers we've all been looking for. It has already led to
one very important conclusion that more physicians need to
embrace: the illnesses we've been discussing may remain unexplained, but they are no more unreal than they are invisible.

## Hope for the Future

Let me now lay out for you some of the treatments that are in the
pipeline.

### Treatments for Orthostatic Intolerance

Orthostatic intolerance means feeling sick when you are on your
feet. Current methods for treating this problem are not very specific, and mainly act by trying to expand your blood volume. You
can do this by drinking at least eight large glasses of fluid a day
and by using salt freely. (Don't do either of these, though, if you
have any evidence of high blood pressure.) Sometimes medicines
can be added to either expand blood volume even more, or else
constrict the blood vessels. In addition, gentle physical conditioning—like toe rises to strengthen the calves or crunches to improve
abdominal muscle strength—can help pump blood back up to the
heart during standing. Medically prescribed Jobst support stock-
ings may also help, especially full tights that cover both your legs
and abdomen. They come in different leg tightnesses; patients with
orthostatic intolerance should try the firmest compression—30 to
40 mm, as ordered by your doctor.

Scientists at the University of Miami received federal funding
to test a different means of expanding blood volume using a

pharmaceutical approach—injection of a hormone, erythropoietin, that regulates red blood cell synthesis. Giving this hormone increases the numbers of red blood cells in the body and thus expands blood volume. The prediction for the project was that this treatment would relieve symptoms of CFS as well as those of orthostatic intolerance in CFS patients who start out with a low blood volume. Preliminary results from the Miami group confirmed that the drug expanded blood volume in those who started out on the low side and also improved a patient's ability to stand for prolonged periods of time. But CFS symptoms did not improve. This was disappointing, but unfortunately, that's the way research works. Your ideas don't always pan out. Some other way of expanding blood volume may work. Dr. David Bell gives some patients with orthostatic intolerance a daily infusion with up to two pints of saline solution. He's done this over long periods of time and strongly believes this treatment can work. The treatment certainly is simple, but it requires a chronically implanted catheter, and these can get infected.

## Drug Trials at Our Center

We are doing a number of potentially important therapeutic trials in my clinical and research group. The first has to do with the drug Xyrem, which I discussed in chapter 7. While there has been one double-blind placebo-controlled trial of this sleep-inducing drug in FM patients, no one has studied what it will do for chronic fatigue. I expect that the drug will relieve the feeling of awakening unrefreshed after a night's sleep. That trial should be underway at the time this book appears in print.

A second path we're pursuing has to do with my ideas concerning the drug selegeline. In chapter 7, I mentioned that the drug given orally in rather low doses showed a slight but positive therapeutic effect. I would expect that giving the drug in higher concentrations may work even better. The availability of a transdermal form of the drug allows this testing to be possible. Whereas high doses of the drug taken by mouth expose patients to the risk of the toxic "cheese effect," this risk is dramatically lessened in the transdermal preparation. Currently the only FDA-approved indication for this preparation is depression, but this drug is much more expensive than other antidepressant drugs available. So your insurance company will balk at paying for this drug, but it may be possible if you have both depression and CFS or FM. If you fall into this group, you should discuss the possibility of this treatment with your doctor. We know your depression will improve; my hope is that your medical symptoms will too. Obviously the best way to learn this is via an appropriate clinical trial. This depends on the interest of the pharmaceutical company. I am currently testing those waters.

## A Device Instead of a Drug

If you think back to the discussions in chapter 7 of the way I treat pain, you will see that treatments for pain often consist of drugs with antidepressant properties and others that treat epilepsy. Although depression and pain can be related, there is no other seeming relation between pain and epilepsy—except for the success of a common group of drugs in both conditions. That is the start of a story about vagal nerve stimulation. The vagus nerve is part of the autonomic nervous system. This particular autonomic nerve carries information from the brain to the heart and stomach and intestines and from those organs back up to brain. It is the parasympathetic branch of the autonomic system that is involved in turning off the fight-or-flight response, moving the body back and forth from a state of alert to one of calm. Vagal nerve stimulation (VNS) is FDA-approved to treat epilepsy when that condition continues, despite good medical treatment. No drug is specific enough to activate only one nerve, so VNS is done by a device.

The story of VNS is fascinating because it is another illustration of how medicine often advances via serendipity. When people with severe epilepsy underwent VNS, an interesting side effect was noted: those with depression felt less depressed. The company that makes the stimulator then adapted the same tactic to target depression that they had used with epilepsy. Since they had tried VNS therapy with patients whose seizures continued despite the proper use of drugs, they did the same with patients whose depression continued despite adequate medication. An international trial showed that VNS is effective, and now the FDA has approved it for treatment-resistant depression—not its original intent, of course, but a great development. Had the device never been used for epilepsy, no one would have dreamed that stimulating the vagus nerve would relieve depression.

But the serendipity continues. Some research on animal test subjects seemed to indicate less pain during VNS. In addition, studies on patients undergoing VNS as a treatment for epilepsy noted a reduction in a different medical problem, namely migraine headaches, as well as learning that stimuli that had been painful in the past no longer were. All these results seemed to be pointing to a brain mechanism that somehow tied epilepsy, depression, and pain together via a brain system that could be damped by VNS.

The fact that people reported less pain during VNS suggested that the treatment reduced the brain sensitization that I had mentioned earlier. This line of thinking led my associate and wife, Dr. Gudrun Lange, to propose doing a preliminary study of VNS to relieve FM pain. That proposal was funded last year, and it has taken her one entire year to get over the various regulatory barriers to allow her team to implant this stimulation package into some FM patients. Specifically, she had to get agreement about all the steps needed to do such a study from the FDA and our own Human Studies Review Board. Approval had to come from one group at a time, so the approval process was long.

Despite those delays, the project is moving ahead, and we implanted our first VNS stimulator in April 2007. Our group at the New Jersey Medical School has a lot of experience in implanting and using these stimulators for patients with epilepsy. Moving to FM is what is novel. We are only considering the treatment for FM patients who continue to have a substantial amount of pain despite treatment with a pain-relieving antidepressant and at least two antiepileptic drugs. Implanting VNS is pretty much the same as putting in a cardiac pacemaker, but a lot less dangerous since we don't go anywhere near the heart. A battery pack strong enough to last a decade is placed under the skin, beneath the clavicle or under a muscle on the side of the chest, while the actual stimulating electrode is placed around the left vagus nerve. This lies to the side of the artery you could feel with your fingers earlier in this chapter.

FM patients are sensitive to painful stimuli, so one purpose of Dr. Lange's study is to determine if FM patients undergoing VNS stimulation are bothered by side effects more than the other patient groups. These side effects could include voice alteration, hoarseness, cough, headache, and feeling short of breath. Since these side effects tend to disappear over time for patients receiving VNS for epilepsy, I expect that they won't be a barrier to the potential use of VNS to reduce FM pain. If this initial study shows that FM patients have no more trouble with VNS than patients with depression, Dr. Lange will mount a larger study to test the efficacy of VNS in treating FM. I am expecting this to happen. And of course, the side benefit of her study will be to prove that FM pain is in the brain and can be reduced without drugs.

## Keeping Up with Clinical Trials

The status of the NIH-approved clinical trial I just described can be followed at a government Web site, www.clinicaltrials.gov. This site plus another one, www.centerwatch.com, track ongoing clinical trials that are initiated by researchers like me. Of the dozens of trials listed, one is for a drug in the same class as Cymbalta but with no proven antidepressant effect. Treatment with this drug, milnacipran, reduced pain and other FM symptoms. The company manufacturing the drug should be moving toward obtaining FDA approval to bring it to market soon. I think approval of this drug will act as a major incentive for other drug companies looking for new markets for new drugs. Nonmalignant pain and fatigue are finally coming into the purview of the pharmaceutical industry. However, drug companies are notoriously secretive about discussing their ideas for treating any disease because of patent issues and their chances of giving leads to another company. It's hard for anyone, including researchers like me, to know what other drugs are already in trials, but the two Web sites listed here may tip you off to new and early studies.

Finally, I wanted to discuss an entirely new class of drugs that is under the investigative microscope for treating fatigue and pain. The drugs act to stimulate one specific serotonin receptor in the brain. The neurotransmitter serotonin is definitely involved in depression, fatigue, and pain, and the specific serotonin receptor targeted by these drugs may primarily influence fatigue and pain. The only one of these drugs available on the American market is ondansetron (Zofran), which is FDA-approved to treat severe nausea and vomiting. One physician reported successfully using it to treat the horrible fatigue that can accompany hepatitis C infection. Zofran, however, is far too expensive and carries too many potentially serious side effects for its use to be considered in a larger context. A group of German psychopharmacologists have been working on another drug from this class, called tropisetron, with potentially fewer side effects. They published a series of studies in 2000 and 2001 suggesting that tropisetron could greatly relieve FM pain. The fact that side effects were still a problem may explain why little else about this drug has appeared in the medical literature since then. However, pharmaceutical companies are now able to "engineer" the drugs they develop so they can hit the target receptors while triggering fewer side effects.

The message I would like you to take home from this section of the book is that illnesses such as FM, CFS, TMD, or IBS are no longer "invisible" to researchers, whether they work in academia or in the pharmaceutical industry. That industry understands that fatigue and pain—whether localized to the mouth or the gut or widespread—are very common and need attention. They are responding to that need, but the process of identifying a molecule that may work and then being sure it does work with limited side effects is a lengthy one. In the meantime, you have this book and your doctors to help you.

# Appendix
# Use of the Freeze-Framer

Freeze-Framer is a device often used by biofeedback therapists, but if you take your time and follow the instructions, you can use it independently. I have no commercial interest in this device, and others like it do exist. I use this one on the advice of several biofeedback therapists whose opinion I value.

Put the pulse detector on a finger and then click Heart Rhythm Display. Select the easiest challenge level and click Start. A few seconds later, you should see your actual heart rate—both as a number and in a graph that moves from right to left, showing your heart rate changing over time. If you don't see this display or if there are a lot of red lines, the pulse sensor is on too loose or your finger is too cold. When your fingers are cold, your blood vessels constrict, making it difficult for the sensor to detect your pulse. If that is the case, just run your hand under warm water for 30 seconds or so. Once you see a good representation of your heart rate, you can follow how well your heart rate tracks your breathing by selecting the box called Coherence Ratio. The goal is to have as high a ratio as possible, which is indicated by a green color. If your heart rate does not cycle from faster to slower with each breath, the link between breathing and heart rate is poor and you will see more red than green. Most people trying Freeze-Framer for the first few times see a lot of red and not a lot of green.

To move things from the red to the green—and from stress to calm—make sure that you can sit in front of your computer without any outside distractions for 7 minutes. Then watch the video display while you slowly breathe in and out. *Slowly* is the operative word. Try to concentrate only on the sound of your breathing and not on other thoughts. As you relax, your breathing rate will slow down. As this happens, you'll start to see the red disappear, and the blue (or even green) will start going up. Put your hand on your tummy as you breathe. You may initially not feel your hand move much, meaning you are breathing mostly through your chest and not through your abdomen. That form of breathing is tiring and is not well coupled with heart rate. As you breathe, try to do it in such a way that you feel your hand move in and out. This abdominal breathing activates the connection between breathing and heart rate. Focusing on positive emotions will help you maintain this peaceful state.

As you achieve change in your breathing, the graph of your heart rate over time may become more variable—going slowly up and then down with each breath—and your coherence values will probably begin to shift from red, to middle levels (blue), and to the tightest link between heart rate and breathing (green). This switch means you are breathing healthily. The critical things that will help you make this change are quiet abdominal breathing and focusing on your breathing alone. If extraneous thoughts pop into your head, refocus on your breathing. The exercise only lasts for a 7-minute period, so this is not hard to do. Sometimes the shift from poor to high coherence between heart and breathing can be helped by exhaling a bit more air at the end of each breath. But just concentrate on quiet breathing with no distracting thoughts in your mind.

Freeze-Framer sums up how well you are doing in something called an *accumulated coherence score*. As the link between your heart and breathing gets better and better (a lot of green, perhaps a bit of blue, and not much red), the program will tell you that you are in *the zone*. This indicates good coupling between heart rate and breathing, which leads to your feeling less stressed. Try to increase the amount of this kind of healthy breathing you do each day by practicing at least twice per day. Eventually, as you get good at this, raise the challenge level at least one notch to Normal. At that point, it might be more fun to move to one of the games provided in the program. To reduce any tendency toward the postural orthostatic syndrome of hyperventilation (POSH), practice this breathing exercise while standing as well as while sitting.

# Notes

## 1. You, Your Symptoms, and Your Doctor

## 2. Tests You Should Expect and Why

## 3. What Doctors Know about Medically Unexplained Illnesses

58    *experienced infectious-type symptoms and fatigue*   Hamilton, 2001
59    *a seven-fold increased risk*   Lucas, 2004
59    *people living near Lake Tahoe*   Buchwald, 1992
60    *for the location of the tender points*   Wolfe, 1990
61    *peaking at 25 percent for women aged sixty to sixty-four*   Bergman, 2001
61    *Rates of FM in Amish women and men*   White, 2003
64    *The group made the decision to diagnose IBS*   Manning, 1978
64    *questionnaire to 1,344 introductory psychology students*   Taub, 1995
65    *use of each of these different clinical case criteria*   Boyce, 2000
65    *One study followed 122 IBS patients*   Hahn, 1998
66    *a greater impairment of normal social functioning*   Gralnek, 2000
66    *One study in Minnesota*   Talley, 1991
68    *One group looked at that exact question*   Aaron, 2000
69    *syndromes are just variations of one another*   Barsky, 1999
69    *those with CFS alone were twice as likely*   Cook, 2005
69    *a severe GI infection increases the risk for developing IBS*   Moss-Morris, 2006
70    *the DePaul researchers*   Taylor, 2001

## 4. When to Seek a Second Opinion and When to See a Specialist
83    *women with CFS feel less stigmatized*   Green, 1999
86    *George Engel, a farsighted physician*   Engel, 1977

## 5. Step One: Getting beyond Depression
101   *We have compared a group of women*   Johnson, 1996
106   *500 patients coming to the doctor*   Bridges, 1985
106   *as the number of medical symptoms went up*   Kroenke, 1997
107   *Patients around the world*   Simon, 1999
107   *rates of alexithymia didn't differ*   Kooiman, 2000
113   *MAOIs are thought to be especially useful*   Quitkin, 2003
116   *Both Beck and Ellis have written books*   Beck, 1985 & Ellis, 1998
116   *Fifty-five percent of patients with depression*   Keller, 2000

## 6. Step Two: Removing Stress and Improving Sleep
118   *risk factor for developing*   Kato, 2006
119   *Hurricane Andrew, the devastating storm*   Lutgendorf, 1995
126   *The Relaxation Response*   Benson, 2000
128   *the Epworth Sleepiness Score*   Johns, 1991
129   *one sleep specialist at the medical school in Stony Brook*   Gold, 2004
130   *In addition, sleep deprivation itself*   Moldofsky, 1976
130   *the average time in bed for a large number of adults*   Lauderdale, 2006
134   *rates of RLS zoom in frequent blood donors*   Silber, 2003
134   *pramipexole (Mirapex)*   Holman, 2005
134   *Sleep-disturbed breathing occurs in up to 20 percent*   Tishler, 2003
135   *many UARS patients are not overweight*   Guilleminault, 2000
135   *People with UARS tend to have lower blood pressure*   Guilleminault, 2001

135  *People with low blood pressure, it turns out,*  Wessely, 1990
136  *one recent study from the medical school at Stony Brook*  Gold, 2003
136  *researchers found a very high rate of UARS in patients*  Gold, 2004

## 7. Step Three: The Role of Drugs in Relieving Pain, Fatigue, and Poor Sleep

141  *One study done many years ago*  Ellis, 1973
142  *evidence of lower than normal levels of this vitamin in the spinal fluid*  Regland, 1997
143  *let alone finding those results with a sugar pill*  Cho, 2005
144  *A recent double-blind placebo-controlled trial*  Blockmans, 2006
145  *An early study showed that it could be useful*  Olson, 2003
145  *I did a trial of selegeline*  Natelson, 1998
146  *These could be an important new avenue for treatment*  Hickie, 2000
146  *reported to reduce severe fatigue is hydrocortisone*  Cleare, 1999
146  *a follow-up trial was not effective*  Blockmans, 2003
147  *a well-done double-blind placebo-controlled trial*  Vollmer-Conna, 1997
147  *very rare in my experience*  Kerr, 2002
147  *a drug called Ampligen*  Strayer, 1994
147  *weekly injections of another immune stimulant*  Zachrisson, 2002
149  *Duloxetine is the first in that class of drugs*  Arnold, 2004
149  *antidepressant treatment can improve some FM symptoms*  O'Malley, 2000
150  *TCAs, as well as a muscle relaxant*  Goldenberg, 1989
151  *This drug is known to have pain-reducing properties*  McLain, 2002
151  *The first one I use is*  Arnold, 2007
151  *pregabalin (Lyrica)*  Crofford, 2005
152  *a painkiller called tramadol (Ultram)*  Bennett, 2003
152  *a need for opiates for some patients*  Kalso, 2003
154  *If the pain disappears during this therapeutic trial*  Clark, 1985
154  *administer additional growth hormone to FM patients*  Bennett, 1998
155  *a similar trial with CFS patients had no effect*  Moorkens, 1998
155  *a drug used to relieve nausea helped reduce fatigue*  Jones, 1999
155  *a drug in this class, tropisetron*  Färber, 2000
155  *preliminary results from an immune active substance*  Russell, 1999
156  *taking 5-HTP three times a day*  Caruso, 1990
157  *Several recent studies show that disturbing sleep*  Moldofsky, 1976 & Lentz, 1999 & Hakkionen, 2001
157  *trial of a drug called sodium oxalate (Xyrem)*  Scharf, 2003

## 8. Step Four: The Integrative Mind-Body Approach

166  *buddy who acts as a coaching partner*  Pesek, 2000
167  *patients who use the buddy system feel stronger*  Pesek, 2000
168  *For example, studies have shown*  Gwee, 1996
168  *Similarly, the presence of fatigue*  Wessely, 1995
168  *Furthermore, focusing on symptoms*  Vercoulen, 1994
170  *CBT, like gentle physical conditioning*  Sharpe, 1996 & Deale, 1997

170   *Furthermore, CBT professionals can concentrate*   Edinger, 2005
170   *CBT is effective in reducing symptoms*   Prins, 2001
170   *improvements you make while using CBT*   Kennedy, 2005
172   *This sense of helplessness can interfere*   Vercoulen, 1994 & Culos-Reed, 2000
175   *This gentle version of aqua-fitness*   Gusi, 2006
177   *Walking to wellness is a method*   Moss-Morris, 2005
178   *The well-known writer Norman Cousins*   Cousins, 1981

## 9. Complementary Treatments

188   *some evidence exists that carnitine*   Plioplys, 1995
188   *One elegant study showed that acetylcarnitine*   Kuratsune, 2002
188   *Moreover, an unblinded trial of carnitine*   Plioplys, 1997
188   *a vitaminlike substance called NADH*   Forsyth, 1999
189   *double-blind study of vitamins and antioxidants*   Brouwers, 2002
190   *One of these studies noted that fatigue*   Martin, 2006
190   *study done on women with neck and shoulder pain*   He, 2004
190   Hypnotherapy *is another potentially useful technique*   Montgomery, 2000
190   *One recent paper reported that hypnotherapy*   Gonsalkorale, 2003
194   *Although tai chi has never been formally tested*   Wang, 2004
195   *Dr. Jim Collins was able to improve*   Priplata, 2003
195   *low blood pressure and fainting during postural challenge*   Bou-Holaigah, 1995
196   *CFS behaves differently in kids*   Stewart, 1998
196   *Because of the existence of POTS in some CFS patients*   Natelson, 2007
197   *due to chronic hyperventilation*   Saisch, 1994
199   *The important thing to emphasize here*   DeGuire, 1996
201   *However, the teachers of this form of yoga*   Shannahoff-Khalsa, 1992
203   *Technique against fatigue and listlessness*   Shannahoff-Khalsa, 1991
204   *health improvements following dietary manipulation*   Haugen, 1991
204   *limited periods of fasting*   Haugen, 1999
204   *Similarly, being on a strict vegan diet*   Kaartinen, 2000
208   The 30-Day Low-Carb Diet Solution   Eades, 2003

## 10. From Complementary Medicine to Quackery

217   *average temperature over a twenty-four-hour period is 98.2 degrees*   Mackowiak, 1992
217   *body temperature in chronic fatigue syndrome (CFS) patients* Hamilos, 1998
218   *placebo-controlled study of vitamins and antioxidants*   Brouwers, 2002
221   *Siberian ginseng for people with CFS*   Hartz, 2004
223   *A double-blind placebo-controlled trial of BioBran*   McDermott, 2006

## 11. Promising Research into the "Invisible Illnesses"

230   *the treatment—one to eradicate EBV*   Straus, 1988
231   *research into chronic fatigue with twins*   Buchwald, 2001 & Hickie, 1999

231   *fatigue and depression did not go hand in hand*   Arnold, 2004

232   *Finally, a group at the University of North Carolina*   Diatchenko, 2005

233   *our own careful review of the immunological literature*   Natelson, 2002

234   *A recent study from the University of Miami*   Siegel, 2006

234   *data existed to indicate that they would have pain too*   Moldofsky, 1976

235   *disrupted sleep with frequent periods of awakening*   Krupp, 1993

236   *One of the first studies I ever did*   DeLuca, 1993

236   *our study found two potentially important results*   Natelson, 2005

237   *The way we check cognitive function*   DeLuca, 1997

237   *abnormalities on brain magnetic resonance imaging*   Lange, 1999

237   *cerebral cortex, was smaller in CFS patients*   De Lange, 2005

238   *My colleagues used functional neuroimaging*   Cook, 2004 & Lange, 2005

239   *and this was not the case*   Gracely, 2002

239   *this is called central sensitization*   Petzke, 2003

239   *interpretation is buttressed by experiments*   Staud, 2001

239   *hypersensitive to the painful stimulus of rectal distention*   Chang, 2000

240   *Instead, the opposite happens:*   Ottenweller, 2001 & LaManca, 2001

241   *abnormal day-to-day activity of the stress hormone cortisol*   Cleare, 2003
      & Korszun, 2002

241   *parasympathetic activity was below normal*   Sisto, 1995

245   *amount of blood the patients' hearts pumped*   Peckerman, 2003

245   *have chronic viral infections of the heart*   Lerner, 1997

245   *did find antibodies to viral building blocks*   Lerner, 2002

245   *The idea that some infectious viral or bacterial agent*   Koelle, 2002 &
      Vernon, 2003

246   *Studies that began at Temple University*   Suhadolnik, 2004

246   *Those patients positive for infection*   Lane, 2003

250   *In addition, studies on patients undergoing VNS*   Kirchner, 2000

251   *Treatment with this drug, milnacipran*   Gendreau, 2005

252   *One physician reported successfully using it*   Jones, 1999

# Bibliography

## 1. You, Your Symptoms, and Your Doctor

Beckman HB, Frankel RM. The effect of physician behavior on the collection of data. *Ann Intern Med* 1993;101:692–6.

Boland BJ, Scheitel SM, Wollan PC, Silverstein MD. Patient-physician agreement on reasons for ambulatory general medical examinations. *Mayo Clin Proc* 1998;73(2):109–17.

Kroenke K, Mangelsdorff AD. Common symptoms in ambulatory care: incidence, evaluation, therapy, and outcome. *Am J Med* 1989;86(3):262–6.

Kroenke K, Spitzer RL. Gender differences in the reporting of physical and somatoform symptoms. *Psychosom Med* 1998;60(2):150–5.

Nimnuan C, Hotopf M, Wessely S. Medically unexplained symptoms: an epidemiological study in seven specialties. *J Psychosom Res* 2001 July;51(1):361–7.

Thompson IM, Pauler DK, Goodman PJ, et al. Prevalence of prostate cancer among men with a prostate-specific antigen level < or = 4.0 ng per milliliter. *N Engl J Med* 2004 May 27;350(22):2239–46.

## 2. Tests You Should Expect and Why

DeLuca J, Johnson SK, Ellis SP, Natelson BH. Cognitive functioning is impaired in chronic fatigue syndrome patients devoid of psychiatric disease. *J Neurol Neurosurg Psychiatry* 1997;62:151–5.

Padgett DA, Hotchkiss AK, Pyter LM, et al. Epstein-Barr virus-encoded dUTPase modulates immune function and induces sickness behavior in mice. *J Med Virol* 2004 November;74(3):442–8.

Pamuk ON, Cakir N. The frequency of thyroid antibodies in fibromyalgia patients and their relationship with symptoms. *Clin Rheumatol* 2007;26(1):55–9.

Rivera J, De Diego A, Trinchet M, Monforte G. Fibromyalgia-associated hepatitis C virus infection. *Br J Rheumatol* 1997;36(9):981–5.

Simini B. Patients' perception of pain with spinal, intramuscular, and venous injections. *Lancet* 2000;355:1076.

Sirois DA, Natelson B. Clinicopathological findings consistent with primary Sjögren's syndrome in a subset of patients diagnosed with chronic fatigue syndrome: preliminary observations. *J Rheumatol* 2001 January;28(1):126–31.

## 3. What Doctors Know about Medically Unexplained Illnesses

Aaron LA, Burke MM, Buchwald D. Overlapping conditions among patients with chronic fatigue syndrome, fibromyalgia, and temporomandibular disorder. *Arch Intern Med* 2000;160:221–7.

Barsky AJ, Borus JF. Functional somatic syndromes. *Ann Intern Med* 1999 June 1;130(11):910–21.

Bergman S, Herrström P, Högström K, Petersson IF, Svensson B, Jacobsson LTH. Chronic musculoskeletal pain, prevalence rates, and sociodemographic associations in a Swedish population study. *J Rheumatol* 2001 June;28(6):1369–77.

Boyce PM, Koloski NA, Talley NJ. Irritable bowel syndrome according to varying diagnostic criteria: are the new Rome II criteria unnecessarily restrictive for research and practice? *Am J Gastroenterol* 2000;95:3176–83.

Buchwald D, Cheney PR, Peterson DL, et al. A chronic illness characterized by fatigue, neurologic and immunologic disorders, and active human herpesvirus type 6 infection. *Ann Intern Med* 1992;116:103–13.

Cook DB, Nagelkirk PR, Peckerman A, Poluri A, Mores J, Natelson BH. Exercise and cognitive performance in Chronic Fatigue Syndrome. *Med Sci Sports Exerc* 2005;37(9):1460–7.

Gralnek IM, Hays RD, Kilbourne A, Naliboff B, Mayer EA. The impact of irritable bowel syndrome on health-related quality of life. *Gastroenterology* 2000 September;119(3):654–60.

Hahn B, Watson M, Yan S, Gunput D, Heuijerjans J. Irritable bowel syndrome symptom patterns: frequency, duration, and severity. *Dig Dis Sci* 1998 December;43(12):2715–8.

Hamilton WT, Hall GH, Round AP. Frequency of attendance in general practice and symptoms before development of chronic fatigue syndrome: a case-control study. *Br J Gen Pract* 2001;51:553–8.

Hotopf M, Noah N, Wessely S. Chronic fatigue and minor psychiatric morbidity after viral meningitis: A controlled study. *J Neurol Neurosurg Psychiatry* 1996;60(5):504–9.

Jason LA, Richman JA, Rademaker AW, et al. A community-based study of chronic fatigue syndrome. *Arch Intern Med* 1999;159:2129–37.

Jason LA, Taylor RR. Applying cluster analysis to define a typology of chronic fatigue syndrome in a medically-evaluated, random community sample. *Psychol Hlth* 2002;1:1–15.

Jason LA, Taylor RR, Kennedy CL, et al. Chronic fatigue syndrome: Symptom subtypes in a community based sample. *Women & Health* 2003;37(1):1–13.

Johnson SK, DeLuca J, Natelson BH. Assessing somatization disorder in the chronic fatigue syndrome. *Psychosom Med* 1996;58(1):50–7.

Lucas KE, Rowe PC, Coresh J, Klag MJ, Meoni LA, Ford DE. Prospective association between hypotension and idiopathic chronic fatigue. *J Hypertens* 2004 April;22(4):691–5.

Manning AP, Thompson WG, Heaton KW, et al. Towards positive diagnosis of the irritable bowel. *BMJ* 1978;2:653–4.

Moss-Morris R, Spence M. To "lump" or to "split" the functional somatic syndromes: can infectious and emotional risk factors differentiate between the onset of chronic fatigue syndrome and irritable bowel syndrome? *Psychosom Med* 2006 May;68(3):463–9.

Solomon L, Reeves WC. Factors influencing the diagnosis of chronic fatigue syndrome. *Arch Intern Med* 2004 November 8;164(20):2241–5.

Swartz M, Landerman R, George L, Blazer D, Escobar J. Somatization disorder. In: Robins LN, Regier D, editors. *Psychiatric Disorders in America*. New York: Free Press, 1991, pp. 220–57.

Talley NJ, Zinsmeister AR, Van Dyke C, Melton LJ, III. Epidemiology of colonic symptoms and the irritable bowel syndrome. *Gastroenterology* 1991;101:927–34.

Taub E, Cuevas JL, Cook EW, III, Crowell M, Whitehead WE. Irritable bowel syndrome defined by factor analysis: gender and race comparisons. *Dig Dis Sci* 1995;40(12):2647–55.

Taylor RR, Jason LA, Schoeny ME. Evaluating latent variable models of functional somatic distress in a community-based sample. *J Ment Health* 2001;10(3):335–49.

White KP, Thompson J. Fibromyalgia syndrome in an Amish community: a controlled study to determine disease and symptom prevalence. *J Rheumatol* 2003 August;30(8):1835–40.

White PD, Thomas JM, Amess J, et al. Incidence, risk and prognosis of acute and chronic fatigue syndromes and psychiatric disorders after glandular fever. *Br J Psychiatry* 1998 December;173(6):475–81.

Wolfe F, Smythe HA, Yunus MB, et al. The American College of Rheumatology 1990 criteria for the classification of fibromyalgia: report of the Multicenter Criteria Committee. *Arthritis Rheum* 1990;33:160–72.

## 4. When to Seek a Second Opinion and When to See a Specialist

Engel GL. The need for a new medical model: a challenge for biomedicine. *Science* 1977 April 8;196(4286):129–36.

Green J, Romei J, Natelson BH. Stigma and chronic fatigue syndrome. *J Chr Fatigue Syndr* 1999;5(2):63–75.

## 5. Step One: Getting beyond Depression

Beck AT, Emery G. *Anxiety Disorders and Phobias: A Cognitive Perspective*. New York: Basic Books, 1985.

Bridges KW, Goldberg DP. Somatic presentation of DSM III psychiatric disorders in primary care. *J Psychosom Res* 1985;29(6):563–9.

Ellis A. *A Guide to Rational Living*, 3rd ed. North Hollywood, CA: Wilshire Book Co., 1998.

Johnson SK, DeLuca J, Natelson BH. Depression in fatiguing illness: comparing patients with chronic fatigue syndrome, multiple sclerosis and depression. *J Affective Disord* 1996;39(1):21–30.

Keller MB, McCullough JP, Klein DN, et al. A comparison of nefazodone, the cognitive behavioral analysis system of psychotherapy, and their combination for the treatment of chronic depression. *N Engl J Med* 2000;342(20):1462–70.

Kooiman CG, Bolk JH, Brand R, Trijsburg RW, Rooijmans HGM. Is alexithymia a risk factor for unexplained physical symptoms in general medical outpatients? *Psychosom Med* 2000 November;62(6):768–78.

Kroenke K, Jackson JL, Chamberlin J. Depressive and anxiety disorders in patients presenting with physical complaints: clinical predictors and outcome. *Am J Med* 1997;103(5):339–47.

Quitkin FM, McGrath PJ, Stewart JW, Klein DF. Columbia atypical depression: a subgroup of depressives with better response to MAOI than to tricylic antidepressants or placebo. *Br J Psychiatry* 2003 April;163(suppl 21):30–4.

Simon GE, VonKorff M, Piccinelli M, Fullerton C, Ormel J. An international study of the relation between somatic symptoms and depression. *N Engl J Med* 1999;341(18):1329–35.

## 6. Step Two: Removing Stress and Improving Sleep

Benson H, Klipper MZ. *The Relaxation Response.* New York: HarperCollins, 2000.

Gold AR, Dipalo F, Gold MS, Broderick J. Inspiratory airflow dynamics during sleep in women with fibromyalgia. *Sleep* 2004 May 1;27(3):459–66.

Gold AR, Dipalo F, Gold MS, O'Hearn D. The symptoms and signs of upper airway resistance syndrome: a link to the functional somatic syndromes. *Chest* 2003 January;123(1):87–95.

Guilleminault C, Faul JL, Stoohs R. Sleep-disordered breathing and hypotension. *Am J Respir Crit Care Med* 2001 October 1;164(7):1242–7.

Guilleminault C, Kim YD, Palombini L, Li K, Powell N. Upper airway resistance syndrome and its treatment. *Sleep* 2000 June 15;23:S197–S200.

Holman AJ, Myers RR. A randomized, double-blind, placebo-controlled trial of pramipexole, a dopamine agonist, in patients with fibromyalgia receiving concomitant medications. *Arthritis Rheum* 2005 August;52(8):2495–505.

Johns MW. A new method for measuring daytime sleepiness: the Epworth sleepiness scale. *Sleep* 1991;14:540–5.

Kato K, Sullivan PF, Evengård B, Pedersen N. Premorbid predictors of chronic fatigue. *Arch Gen Psychiatry* 2006; 63:1267–72.

Lauderdale DS, Knutson KL, Yan LL, et al. Objectively measured sleep characteristics among early-middle-aged adults: the CARDIA study. *Am J Epidemiol* 2006 July 1;164(1):5–16.

Lutgendorf SK, Antoni MH, Ironson G, et al. Physical symptoms of chronic fatigue syndrome are exacerbated by the stress of Hurricane Andrew. *Psychosom Med* 1995;57:310–23.

Moldofsky H, Scarisbrick P. Induction of neurasthenic musculoskeletal pain syndrome by selective sleep stage deprivation. *Psychosom Med* 1976;38(1):35–44.

Silber MH, Richardson JW. Multiple blood donations associated with iron deficiency in patients with restless leg syndrome. *Mayo Clin Proc* 2003;78:52–4.

Tishler PV, Larkin EK, Schluchter MD, Redline S. Incidence of sleep-disordered breathing in an urban adult population: the relative importance of risk factors in the development of sleep-disordered breathing. *JAMA* 2003 May 7;289 (17):2230–7.

Wessely S, Nickson J, Cox B. Symptoms of low blood pressure: a population study. *BMJ* 1990;301:362–5.

## 7. Step Three: The Role of Drugs in Relieving Pain, Fatigue, and Poor Sleep

Arnold LM, Lu YL, Crofford LJ, et al. A double-blind, multicenter trial comparing duloxetine with placebo in the treatment of fibromyalgia patients with or without major depressive disorder. *Arthritis Rheum* 2004 September; 50(9):2974–84.

Arnold LM, Goldenberg DL, Stanford SB, et al. Gabapentin in the treatment of fibromyalgia. *Arthritis Rheum* 2007 April; 56(4):1336–44.

Bennett RA, Kamin M, Karim R, Rosenthal N. Tramadol and acetaminophen combination tablets in the treatment of fibromyalgia pain: a double-blind, randomized, placebo-controlled study. *Am J Med* 2003 May;114(7):537–45.

Bennett RM, Clark SC, Walczyk J. A randomized, double-blind, placebo-controlled study of growth hormone in the treatment of fibromyalgia. *Am J Med* 1998;104(3):227–31.

Blockmans D, Persoons P, Van Houdenhove B, Lejeune M, Bobbaers H. Combination therapy with hydrocortisone and fludrocortisone does not improve symptoms in chronic fatigue syndrome: a randomized, placebo-controlled, double-blind crossover study. *Am J Med* 2003;114:736–41.

Blockmans D, Persoons P, Van HB, Bobbaers H. Does methylphenidate reduce the symptoms of chronic fatigue syndrome? *Am J Med* 2006 February;119(2): 167–30.

Caruso I, Sarzi-Puttini P, Cazzola M, Azzolini V. Double-blind study of 5-hydroxytryptophan versus placebo in the treatment of primary fibromyalgia syndrome. *J Int Med Res* 1990;18:201–9.

Cho HJ, Hotopf M, Wessely S. The placebo response in the treatment of chronic fatigue syndrome: a systematic review and meta-analysis. *Psychosom Med* 2005 March;67(2):301–13.

Clark S, Tindall E, Bennett RM. A double-blind crossover tiral of prednisone versus placebo in the treatment of fibrositis. *J Rheumatol* 1985;12(5):980–3.

Cleare AJ, Heap E, Malhi GS, Wessely S, O'Keane V, Miell J. Low-dose hydrocortisone in chronic fatigue syndrome: a randomised crossover trial. *Lancet* 1999 February 6;353(9151):455–8.

Crofford LJ, Rowbotham MC, Mease PJ, et al. Pregabalin for the treatment of fibromyalgia syndrome: results of a randomized, double-blind, placebo-controlled trial. *Arthritis Rheum* 2005 April;52(4):1264–73.

Ellis FR, Nasser S. A pilot study of vitamin B12 in the treatment of tiredness. *Br J Nutr* 1973;30:277–83.

Färber L, Stratz T, Brückle W, et al. Efficacy and tolerability of tropisetron in primary fibromyalgia: a highly selective and competitive 5-HT3 receptor antagonist. *Scand J Rheumatol* 2000;29:49–54.

Goldenberg DL. A review of the role of tricyclic medications in the treatment of fibromyalgia syndrome. *J Rheumatol* 1989;16 Suppl. 19:137–9.

Hakkionen S, Alloui A, Gross A, Eschallier A, Dubray C. The effects of total sleep deprivation, selective sleep interruption and sleep recovery on pain tolerance in healthy subjects. *J Sleep Res* 2001;10:35–42.

Hickie IB, Wilson AJ, Wright JM, Bennett BK, Wakefield D, Lloyd AR. A randomized, double-blind, placebo-controlled trial of moclobemide in patients with chronic fatigue syndrome. *J Clin Psychiatry* 2000 August;61(9):643–8.

Jones EA. Relief from profound fatigue associated with chronic liver disease by long-term ondansetron therapy. *Lancet* 1999 July 31;354(9176):397.

Kalso E, Allan L, Dellemijn PL, et al. Recommendations for using opioids in chronic non-cancer pain. *Eur J Pain* 2003;7(5):381–6.

Kerr JR, Bracewell J, Laing I, et al. Chronic fatigue syndrome and arthraliga following parvovirus B19 infection. *J Rheumatol* 2002 March;29(3):595–602.

Lentz MJ, Landis CA, Rothermel J, Shaver JL. Effects of selective slow wave sleep disruption on musculoskeletal pain and fatigue in middle aged women. *J Rheumatol* 1999;26(7):1586–92.

McLain D. An open label dose finding trial of tizanidine [Zanaflex] for treatment of fibromyalgia. *J Musculoskel Pain* 2002;10(4):7–18.

Moldofsky H, Scarisbrick P. Induction of neurasthenic musculoskeletal pain syndrome by selective sleep stage deprivation. *Psychosom Med* 1976;38(1):35–44.

Moorkens G, Wynants H, Abs R. Effect of growth hormone treatment in chronic fatigue syndrome: a preliminary study. *Growth Horm* IGF Res 1998;8:131–3.

Natelson BH, Cheu J, Hill N, et al. Single blind, placebo-phase in trial of two escalating doses of selegiline in the chronic fatigue syndrome. *Neuropsychobiology* 1998; 37:150–4.

O'Malley PG, Balden E, Tomkins G, Santoro J, Kroenke K, Jackson JL. Treatment of fibromyalgia with antidepressants: a meta-analysis. *J Gen Intern Med* 2000; 15:659–66.

Olson LG, Ambrogetti A, Sutherland DC. A pilot randomized controlled trial of dexamphetamine in patients with Chronic Fatigue Syndrome. *Psychosomatics* 2003; 44(1):38–43.

Regland B, Andersson M, Abrahamsson L, Bagby J, Dyrehag LE, Gottfries CG. Increased concentrations of homocysteine in the cerebrospinal fluid in patients with fibromyalgia and chronic fatigue syndrome. *Scand J Rheumatol* 1997; 26:301.

Russell IJ, Michalek JE, Kang YK, Richards AB. Reduction of morning stiffness and improvement in physical function in fibromyalgia syndrome patients treated sublingually with low doses of human interferon-α. *J Interferon Cytokine Res* 1999 August;19(8):961–8.

Scharf MB, Baumann M, Berkowitz DV. The effects of sodium oxybate on clinical symptoms and sleep patterns in patients with fibromyalgia. *J Rheumatol* 2003 May;30(5):1070–4.

Strayer DR, Carter WA, Brodsky I, et al. A controlled clinical trial with a specifically configured RNA drug, poly(I)•poly(C12U), in chronic fatigue syndrome. *Clin Infect* Dis 1994;18 Suppl. 1:S88–S95.

Vollmer-Conna U, Hickie I, Hadzi-Pavlovic D, et al. Intravenous immunoglobulin is ineffective in the treatment of patients with chronic fatigue syndrome. *Am J Med* 1997;103(1):38–43.

Zachrisson O, Regland B, Jahreskog M, Jonsson M, Kron M, Gottfries C-G. Treatment with staphylococcus toxoid in fibromyalgia/chronic fatigue syndrome: a randomized controlled trial. *Eur J Pain* 2002;6:455–66.

## 8. Step Four: The Integrative Mind-Body Approach

Cousins N. *Anatomy of an Illness as Perceived by the Patient*. New York: Bantam Books, 1981.

Culos-Reed SN, Brawley LR. Fibromyalgia, physical activity, and daily functioning: the importance of efficacy and health-related quality of life. *Arthritis Care Res* 2000 December;13(6):343–51.

Deale A, Chalder T, Marks I, Wessely S. Cognitive behavior therapy for chronic fatigue syndrome: a randomized controlled trial. *Am J Psychiatry* 1997; 154(3):408–14.

Edinger JD, Wohlgemuth WK, Krystal AD, Rice JR. Behavioral insomnia therapy for fibromyalgia patients: a randomized clinical trial. *Arch Intern Med* 2005 November 28;165(21):2527–35.

Gusi N, Tomas-Carus P, Hakkinen A, Hakkinen K, Ortega-Alonso A. Exercise in waist-high warm water decreases pain and improves health-related quality of life and strength in the lower extremities in women with fibromyalgia. *Arthritis Rheum* 2006 February 15;55(1):66–73.

Gwee KA, Graham JC, McKendrick MW, et al. Psychometric scores and persistence of irritable bowel after infectious diarrhoea. *Lancet* 1996;347(8995): 150–3.

Kennedy T, Jones R, Darnley S, Seed P, Wessely S, Chalder T. Cognitive behaviour therapy in addition to antispasmodic treatment for irritable bowel syndrome in primary care: randomised controlled trial. *BMJ* 2005 August 20;331(7514): 435.

Moss-Morris R, Sharon C, Tobin R, Baldi JC. A randomized controlled graded exercise trial for chronic fatigue syndrome: outcomes and mechanisms of change. *J Health Psychol* 2005 March;10(2):245–59.

Pesek JR, Jason LA, Taylor RR. An empirical investigation of the envelope theory. *J Hum Behav Soc Environ* 2000;3:59–77.

Prins JB, Bleijenberg G, Bazelmans E, et al. Cognitive behaviour therapy for chronic fatigue syndrome: a multicentre randomised controlled trial. *Lancet* 2001 March 17;357(9259):841–7.

Sharpe M, Hawton K, Simkin S, et al. Cognitive behaviour therapy for the chronic fatigue syndrome: a randomised controlled trial. *BMJ* 1996;312(7022):22–6.

Vercoulen JHMM, Swanink CMA, Fennis JFM, Galama JMD, Van der Meer JWM, Bleijenberg G. Dimensional assessment of chronic fatigue syndrome. *J Psychosom Res* 1994;38(5):383–92.

Wessely S, Chalder T, Hirsch S, Pawlikowska T, Wallace P, Wright DJM. Postinfectious fatigue: prospective cohort study in primary care. *Lancet* 1995;345: 1333–8.

## 9. Complementary Treatments

Bou-Holaigah I, Rowe PC, Kan J, Calkins H. The relationship between neurally mediated hypotension and the chronic fatigue syndrome. *JAMA* 1995;274 (12):961–7.

Brouwers PM, van der Werf S, Bleijenberg G, Van der Zee L, van der Meer JWM. The effect of a polynutrient supplement on fatigue and physical activity of patients with chronic fatigue syndrome: a double-blind randomized controlled trial. *Q J Med* 2002;95:677–83.

DeGuire S, Gevirtz R, Hawkinson D, Dixon K. Breathing retraining: a three-year follow-up study of treatment for hyperventilation syndrome and associated functional cardiac symptoms. *Biofeedback Self-Reg* 1996;21(2):191–8.

Eades MR, Eades MD. *The 30-Day Low-Carb Diet Solution*. New York: John Wiley & Sons, 2003.

Forsyth LM, Preuss HG, MacDowell AL, Chiazze L, Jr., Birkmayer GD, Bellanti JA. Therapeutic effects of oral NADH on the symptoms of patients with chronic fatigue syndrome. *Ann Allergy Asthma Immunol* 1999 February;82(2):185–91.

Gonsalkorale WM, Miller V, Afzal A, Whorwell PJ. Long term benefits of hypnotherapy for irritable bowel syndrome. *Gut* 2003 November;52(11):1623–9.

Haugen M, Fraser D, Forre O. Diet therapy for the patient with rheumatoid arthritis? *Rheumatology* (Oxford) 1999 November;38(11):1039–44.

Haugen M, Kjeldsen-Kragh J, Nordvag BY, Forre O. Diet and disease symptoms in rheumatic diseases: results of a questionnaire based survey. *Clin Rheumatol* 1991 December;10(4):401–7.

He D, Veiersted KB, Høstmark AT, Medbø JI. Effect of acupuncture treatment on chronic neck and shoulder pain in sedentary female workers: a 6-month and 3-year follow-up study. *Pain* 2004;109:299–307.

Kaartinen K, Lammi K, Hypen M, Nenonen M, Hänninen O, Rauma AL. Vegan diet alleviates fibromyalgia symptoms. *Scand J Rheumatol* 2000;29(5):308–13.

Kuratsune H, Yamaguti K, Lindh G, et al. Brain regions involved in fatigue sensation: reduced acetylcarnitine uptake into the brain. *Neuroimage* 2002 November;17(3):1256–65.

Martin DP, Sletten CD, Williams BA, Berger IH. Improvement in fibromyalgia symptoms with acupuncture: results of a randomized controlled trial. *Mayo Clin Proc* 2006 June;81(6):749–57.

Montgomery GH, DuHamel KN, Redd WH. A meta-analysis of hypnotically induced analgesia: how effective is hypnosis? *Int J Clin Exp Hypn* 2000 April;48(2):138–53.

Natelson BH, Intriligator R, Chandler HK, Cherniack NS, Stewart JM. Hypocapnia is a biological marker for orthostatic intolerance. *Dynamic Med.* 2007;6(1):2.

Plioplys AV, Plioplys S. Serum levels of carnitine in chronic fatigue syndrome: clinical correlates. *Neuropsychobiology* 1995;32(3):132–8.

Plioplys AV, Plioplys S. Amantadine and L-carnitine treatment of chronic fatigue syndrome. *Neuropsychobiology* 1997;35(1):16–23.

Priplata AA, Niemi JB, Harry JD, Lipsitz LA, Collins JJ. Vibrating insoles and balance control in elderly people. *Lancet* 2003 October 4;362(9390):1123–4.

Saisch SGN, Deale A, Gardner WN, Wessely S. Hyperventilation and chronic fatigue syndrome. *Q J Med* 1994;87:63–7.

Shannahoff-Khalsa D, Bhajan Y. The healing power of sound: techniques from yogic medicine. In: Spintge R, Droh R, editors. *MusicMedicine.*St. Louis, MO: MMB Music, 1992, pp. 179–93.

Shannahoff-Khalsa D . Stress technology medicine: a new paradigm for stress and considerations for self-regulation. In: Brown M, Rivier C, Koob G, editors. *Stress: Neurobiology and Neuroendocrinology.* New York: Marcel Dekker, 1991. pp. 647–86.

Stewart J, Weldon A, Arlievsky N, Li K, Munoz J. Neurally mediated hypotension and autonomic dysfunction measured by heart rate variability during head-up tilt testing in children with chronic fatigue syndrome. *Clin Auton Res* 1998 August;8(4):221–30.

Wang C, Collet JP, Lau J. The effect of Tai Chi on health outcomes in patients with chronic conditions: a systematic review. *Arch Intern Med* 2004 March 8;164(5):493–501.

## 10. From Complementary Medicine to Quackery

Brouwers PM, van der Werf S, Bleijenberg G, Van der Zee L, van der Meer JWM. The effect of a polynutrient supplement on fatigue and physical activity of patients with chronic fatigue syndrome: a double-blind randomized controlled trial. *Q J Med* 2002;95:677–83.

Hamilos DL, Nutter D, Gershtenson J, et al. Core body temperature is normal in chronic fatigue syndrome. *Biol Psychiatry* 1998;43(4):293–302.

Hartz AJ, Bentler S, Noyes R, et al. Randomized controlled trial of Siberian ginseng for chronic fatigue. *Psychol Med 2004 January;34(1):51–61.*

Mackowiak PA, Wasserman SS, Levine MM. A critical appraisal of 98.6°F, the upper limit of the normal body temperature, and other legacies of Carl Reinhold August Wunderlich. *JAMA* 1992;268:1578–80.

McDermott C, Richards SCM, Thomas PW, Montgomery J, Lewith G. A placebo-controlled, double-blind, randomized controlled trial of a natural killer cell stimulant (BioBran MGN-3) in chronic fatigue syndrome. *Q J Med* 2006; 99:461–8.

## 11. Promising Research into the "Invisible Illnesses"

Arnold LM, Hudson JI, Hess EV, et al. Family study of fibromyalgia. *Arthritis Rheum* 2004 March;50(3):944–52.

Buchwald D, Herrell R, Ashton S, et al. A twin study of chronic fatigue. *Psychosom Med* 2001 November;63(6):936–43.

Chang L, Mayer EA, Johnson T, FitzGerald LZ, Naliboff B. Differences in somatic perception in female patients with irritable bowel syndrome with and without fibromyalgia. *Pain* 2000 February;84(2-3):297–307.

Cleare AJ. The neuroendocrinology of chronic fatigue syndrome. *Endocr Rev* 2003;24(2):236–52.

Cook DB, Lange G, Ciccone DS, Liu WC, Steffener J, Natelson BH. Functional imaging of pain in patients with primary fibromyalgia. *J Rheumatol* 2004 February;31(2):364–78.

De Lange FP, Kalkman JS, Bleijenberg G, Hagoort P, van der Meer JW, Toni I. Gray matter volume reduction in the chronic fatigue syndrome. *Neuroimage* 2005 July 1;26(3):777–81.

DeLuca J, Johnson SK, Ellis SP, Natelson BH. Cognitive functioning is impaired in chronic fatigue syndrome patients devoid of psychiatric disease. *J Neurol Neurosurg Psychiatry* 1997;62:151–5.

DeLuca J, Johnson SK, Natelson BH. Information processing efficiency in chronic fatigue syndrome and multiple sclerosis. *Arch Neurol* 1993;50:301–4.

Diatchenko L, Slade GD, Nackley AG, et al. Genetic basis for individual variations in pain perception and the development of a chronic pain condition. *Hum Mol Genet* 2005 January 1;14(1):135–43.

Gendreau RM, Thorn MD, Gendreau JF, et al. Efficacy of milnacipran in patients with fibromyalgia. *J Rheumatol* 2005 October;32(10):1975–85.

Gracely RH, Petzke F, Wolf JM, Clauw DJ. Functional magnetic resonance imaging evidence of augmented pain processing in fibromyalgia. *Arthritis Rheum* 2002 May;46(5):1333–43.

Hickie I, Kirk K, Martin N. Unique genetic and environmental determinants of prolonged fatigue: a twin study. *Psychol Med* 1999 March;29(2):259–68.

Jones EA. Relief from profound fatigue associated with chronic liver disease by long-term ondansetron therapy. *Lancet* 1999 July 31;354(9176):397.

Kirchner A, Birklein F, Stefan H, Handwerker HO. Left vagus nerve stimulation suppresses experimentally induced pain. *Neurology* 2000 October 24;55(8):1167–71.

Koelle DM, Barcy S, Huang ML, et al. Markers of viral infection in monozygotic twins discordant for chronic fatigue syndrome. *Clin Infect Dis* 2002 September 1;35(5):518–25.

Korszun A, Young EA, Singer K, Carlson NE, Crofford L. Basal circadian cortisol secretion in women with temporomandibular disorders. *J Dent Res* 2002;81(4):279–83.

Krupp LB, Jandorf L, Coyle PK, Mendelson WB. Sleep disturbance in chronic fatigue syndrome. *J Psychosom Res* 1993;37:325–31.

LaManca JJ, Peckerman A, Sisto SA, DeLuca J, Cook S, Natelson BH. Cardiovascular responses of women with chronic fatigue syndrome to stressful cognitive testing before and after strenuous exercise. *Psychosom Med* 2001 September;63(5):756–64.

Lane RJM, Soteriou BA, Zhang H, Archard LC. Enterovirus related metabolic myopathy: a postviral fatigue syndrome. *J Neurol Neurosurg Psychiatry* 2003 October;74(10):1382–6.

Lange G, DeLuca J, Maldjian JA, Lee HJ, Tiersky LA, Natelson BH. Brain MRI abnormalities exist in a subset of patients with chronic fatigue syndrome. *J Neurol Sci* 1999 December 1;171(1):3–7.

Lange G, Steffener J, Bly BM, et al. Chronic fatigue syndrome affects verbal working memory: a BOLD fMRI study. *Neuroimage* 2005;26(2):513–24.

Lerner AM, Beqaj SH, Deeter RG, Fitzgerald JT. IgM serum antibodies to human cytomegalovirus nonstructureal gene products p52 and CM2 are uniquely present in a subset of patients with chronic fatigue syndrome. *In Vivo* 2002; 16:153–60.

Lerner AM, Zervos M, Dworkin HJ, Chang CH, O'Neill W. A unified theory of the cause of chronic fatigue syndrome. *Infect Dis Clin Pract* 1997;6:239–43.

Moldofsky H, Scarisbrick P. Induction of neurasthenic musculoskeletal pain syndrome by selective sleep stage deprivation. *Psychosom Med* 1976;38(1):35–44.

Natelson BH, Haghighi MH, Ponzio NM. Evidence for the presence of immune dysfunction in chronic fatigue syndrome. *Clin Diagn Lab Immunol* 2002 July; 9(4):747–52.

Natelson BH, Tseng C-L, Ottenweller JE. Spinal fluid abnormalities in patients with chronic fatigue syndrome. *Clin Diagn Lab Immunol* 2005; 12(1):53–5.

Ottenweller JE, Sisto SA, McCarty RC, Natelson BH. Hormonal responses to exercise in chronic fatigue syndrome. *Neuropsychobiology* 2001; 43(1):34–41.

Peckerman A, LaManca JJ, Dahl K, Qureishi B, Natelson BH. Abnormal impedance cardiography predicts symptom severity in chronic fatigue syndrome. *Am J Med Sci 2003* April; 326(2):55–60.

Petzke F, Clauw DJ, Ambrose K, Khine A, Gracely RH. Increased pain sensitivity in fibromyalgia: effects of stimulus type and mode of presentation. *Pain* 2003 October; 105(3):403–13.

Siegel SD, Antoni MH, Fletcher MA, Maher K, Segota MC, Klimas N. Impaired natural immunity, cognitive dysfunction, and physical symptoms in patients with chronic fatigue syndrome: preliminary evidence for a subgroup. *J Psychosom Res* 2006 September; 60:559–66.

Sisto S, Tapp WN, Drastal SD, et al. Vagal tone is decreased during paced breathing in patients with the chronic fatigue syndrome. *Clin Auton Res* 1995; 5:139–43.

Staud R, Vierck CJ, Cannon RL, Mauderli AP, Price DD. Abnormal sensitization and temporal summation of second pain (wind-up) in patients with fibromyalgia syndrome. *Pain* 2001 March; 91(1–2):165–75.

Straus SE, Dale JK, Tobi M et al. Acyclovir treatment of the chronic fatigue syndrome. *N Engl J Med* 1988; 319:1692–8.

Suhadolnik RJ, Peterson DL, Reichenbach NL, et al. Clinical and biochemical characteristics differentiating chronic fatigue syndrome from major depression and healthy control populations: relation to dysfunction in the RNase L pathway. *J Chr Fatigue Syndr* 2004; 12(1):5–35.

Vernon SD, Shukla SK, Reeves WC. Absence of Mycoplasma species DNA in chronic fatigue syndrome. *J Med Microbiol* 2003 November; 52(Pt 11):1027–8.

# Index

Note: Drugs are listed under their generic names.